D1708519

The facts behind the fastest-selling medication in history!

FACT: Up to thirty million American men suffer from impotence—nearly 10% of the total population and 23% of all adult males.

FACT: Clinical trials are already under way to see whether Viagra will aid women who have difficulty with vaginal lubrication and reaching orgasm.

FACT: The vicious cycle of anticipatory performance anxiety only compounds male impotency problems, leading to broken hearts, broken marriages, and broken egos.

FACT: Using Viagra means that men can have sex when they want it—even if they're one hundred!

FACT: Hundreds of thousands of couples have already benefited from Viagra—and demand for the drug grows steadily every day.

FACT: No drug should be taken without a full understanding of its effects—and there is no better complete resource available on Viagra than *VIAGRA*.

VIAGRA

A GUIDE TO THE PHENOMENAL POTENCY-PROMOTING DRUG

SUSAN C. VAUGHAN, M.D.

POCKET BOOKS
New York   London   Toronto   Sydney   Tokyo   Singapore

An *Original* Publication of POCKET BOOKS

POCKET BOOKS, a division of Simon & Schuster Inc.
1230 Avenue of the Americas, New York, NY 10020

Copyright © 1998 by Susan C. Vaughan, M.D.

All rights reserved, including the right to reproduce this book or portions thereof in any form whatsoever. For information address Pocket Books, 1230 Avenue of the Americas, New York, NY 10020

ISBN: 0-671-02733-6

First Pocket Books printing June 1998

10 9 8 7 6 5 4 3

POCKET and colophon are registered trademarks of Simon & Schuster Inc.

Printed in the U.S.A.

To all the men and women who will be able to look beyond sexual function and focus on building strong and enduring relationships.

Contents

Contents

PART III: Women and Viagra

VIAGRA

Introduction:
The Bull Market for Viagra

A sports car that's lost its turbocharge."

"The king of the jungle without a roar."

"Power tools without power."

"The Marlboro Man put out to pasture."

These are a few of the images some men use to describe themselves when they suffer from erectile dysfunction, vividly evoking the loss of personal power and the decrease in masculine self-esteem that erectile dysfunction so often produces.

It's no wonder, then, that when Viagra, the new treatment for impotence, hit the shelves in April it sparked a stampede. Men rushed to their doctors' offices and their pharmacies for the hottest new boost to masculinity since the matador, in a scene reminiscent of the running of the bulls in Pamplona. What these men were after was the rebirth of their own virility and sexual stamina. They wanted to feel young and potent again. They wanted to feel like themselves as they used to be. They wanted Viagra, and they wanted it now.

These modern matadors were bullish about the future—the sexual future, to be specific—and with good reason. In clinical trials, Viagra was an effective treatment for impotence in almost 80% of patients who tried it. Perhaps the most bullish of all was Pfizer Pharmaceuticals, makers of Viagra. Viagra is the first-ever oral medication for erectile dysfunction, eliminating the need for the needles past medicines required. It works when a man is sexually stimulated, magnifying the normal process of sexual arousal. Unlike other medications, Viagra will not work without stimulation. So if a man takes Viagra and his partner later declines to have sex, he will not get an erection anyway. Viagra's side effects are minimal—headaches, flushing, stomachaches, and shifts in blue-green color vision being the most noteworthy.

Anticipation of Viagra's release was largely responsible for pushing Pfizer's stock to all-time highs, with an increase of 100% in the year before its FDA approval. It's probably no coincidence that Viagra's release and the Dow's breaking 9,000 happened nearly simultaneously. With Viagra in its veins, the bull market raged on. But as Viagra entered the final stages of FDA approval, some market-watchers grew bearish. Perhaps the claims of Viagra had been oversold. Maybe interest and enthusiasm would fizzle when the drug hit the streets.

The bears were quickly butted aside as Viagra thundered past. In the first two weeks after its release, between April 1 and April 15, 1998, Viagra gained 79% of the market share. That made it the most successful launch of a new drug in pharmaceutical history and the fastest-selling medication in the history of medicine. Pfizer stock jumped over eight dollars a share in one day. Analysts revised their estimates of 1998 Viagra sales from $400 million to $600 million. Doctors wrote almost forty thousand prescriptions in the first week alone. Then, proving that the pen was indeed mighty in the fight against erectile dysfunction, they wrote another forty thousand scripts a day in the second week. One Atlanta urologist, Dr. John Stripling, finally wised up in week two and got a rubber stamp to prescribe the pill after he developed writer's cramp by penning five hundred scripts for Viagra the week before.

Men scoring the scripts scoured the Internet, looking for a pharmacy near them that had the pill in stock. Pfizer salesmen's cars were reportedly broken into as men frantically searched for the hard-to-find hard drug. Overnight the little blue diamond-shaped pills became man's best friend.

Other men went directly to the Web to get the pill in the first place, where some unscrupulous physicians wrote prescriptions after an "on-line" exam. A black market developed overnight, with reports of the pricey ten-dollar pill selling for as much as five times that on the street.

The deafening roar of media attention, the men racing to get it, the reaction of the stock market—everywhere there were signs of the lengths that men would go to in their efforts to restore their sexual equipment to its proper working order.

Yet despite all the commotion about Viagra in the world outside, my office was quiet except for the soft whir of the air conditioner. Just me, Ted, and his problem.

"Sarah's been great about it," Ted said, "and I've been trying to please her anyway, concentrating on her pleasure in bed. But I feel like a failure. I really love my wife, and this basic, fundamental way of showing it is simply not an option anymore. Here I am, only fifty-eight years old and I feel like my sexual life is over. It feels unfair. I know there are things I could be doing to help with _my diabetes, like_ _losing weight,_ but it's hard for me to go to the gym. I look at all those young guys with hard bodies and washboard abs, and all I can think is that they don't have a problem—they're hard in bed as well. Sarah and I are happy. We have a nice home, children we love, everything. I'm doing well at work and so is she. But this problem sometimes seems like it could tear all that apart. In my darkest moments, I imagine her leaving me for a real man. She's been incredibly supportive and reassuring, but sex used to be such an important part of our lives together. Now it's anxiety-producing. I've even started to wonder if all my worries about whether I'll get and keep an erection aren't making my problem worse. I need your help."

Ted looked down, his eyes tracing the floral patterns of my rug the way patients often do when they feel anxious and ashamed. Like many men with erectile dysfunction, he was unused to discussing his problem with anyone. He'd said on the phone that he thought it might be easier to talk about with a woman, but it was clearly very difficult to talk about it at all.

Ted is one of an estimated thirty million men across America who suffer from erectile dysfunction, which is defined as inability to achieve and maintain an erection adequate for penetration during intercourse. Until Viagra, less than 5% of the men who had the problem sought help. Partly this was because the treatments available before Viagra were painful or cumbersome. But clearly much of the issue is that the problem of impotence comes perilously close to threatening a man's image of himself as a man.

In the past, admitting you had erectile dysfunction was a bit like admitting you weren't a real, red-blooded American man after all. It's easy to see why: The OED defines impotence as "want of strength or power to perform anything, utter inability or weakness, helplessness, want of physical power, feebleness of body, complete absence of sexual power." With a definition like that, it's easy to understand why so many men kept quiet. Even within relationships deeply affected by erectile dysfunction, relationships such as Ted and Sarah's, where good communication was the norm, often little was said. Many men and women tiptoed around the subject in the bedroom, uncertain how to broach the topic.

Now Viagra promises to bring all that hiding and secrecy, all that living in silence, to an end.

If you're one of the new stampede already taking Viagra or if you're thinking of putting yourself in the running, this book is for you.

If you're the partner of someone with erectile dysfunction, this book will help you understand the problem, the options, and the psychological ramifications of erectile dysfunction within your relationship as well.

And if you're a woman interested in the latest on Viagra for women, you'll find it right here.

This book will take you step by step through the problem of erectile dysfunction, its solution, and a review of what Viagra may offer women as well. In Part I: The Impotence Problem, we'll take a look at what erectile dysfunction is and where it comes from. In Chapter 1, you'll learn how your penis works, a kind of owner's manual for the manly organ, like the one you have that tells you about your car. Like engine trouble, erectile dysfunction has a wide range of causes. Everything from normal aging to prescription medication, alcohol to atherosclerosis, anxiety to prostate surgery and diabetes to .

bicycle seats can be a culprit. In Chapter 2, you'll see what can go wrong when your penis isn't working properly and how Viagra can help. Because mind matters in controlling erections as well, Chapter 3 will take a look at the psychology of desire and arousal as well as the psychological issues that can interfere with erectile function. Chapter 4 will help you sort out whether the causes of your erectile dysfunction are likely to be physical or psychological or—as Ted astutely noted and is commonly the case—a mixture of both. This chapter will also give you an overview of the evaluation of your erectile dysfunction that your physician will perform, with a detailed description of what medical tests may be necessary. Although some men are bypassing careful medical evaluation in their rush for a cure, knowing why you have erectile dysfunction is important, since some serious systemic illnesses such as diabetes can first be manifest that way.

Once you have a thorough understanding of the problem, we'll turn in Part II to The Viagra Solution. In Chapter 5, you'll hear the hopes and concerns of individuals and couples I've treated as they contemplated Viagra. Their reactions, like the causes of their erectile dysfunctions, run the gamut. In Chapter 6, you'll learn all you need to know about Viagra: how it works, what its side effects are and where they come from, what medicines you can and cannot take with it, the types of erectile dysfunction for which it works best. And you'll hear the first-night kiss-and-tell stories of my patients and explore their physical and psychological reactions to taking Viagra.

Because Viagra doesn't work or isn't right for everybody, in Chapter 7 we'll take a look at alternatives to Viagra, from vacuum pumps and penile implants to vascular surgery and alternative medications, plus we'll see what new treatments are on the horizon to treat erectile dysfunction. So if Viagra doesn't work for you, don't despair; there are alternatives that probably will. Because erectile dysfunction and its treatment extend far beyond the ups and downs of the penis, in Chapter 8 we'll look at what psychotherapy has to offer men with erectile dysfunction and their partners, whether with or without Viagra or an alternative.

Part III: Women and Viagra will take a look at what the drug has done for women. Chapter 9 will examine women's reactions to men's use of the pill, from agonizing psychological concerns to reports of their own ecstasy about their renewed sex lives. Chapter 10 will break new ground by examining the latest on what the pill may have to offer women who suffer from the female version of erectile dysfunction. Clitoral engorgement and vaginal lubrication in women correspond to erection—the engorgement of the penis with blood—in men. So because Viagra increases both clitoral engorgement and vaginal lubrication in women, you'll see why it may help them as well. Lubrication and clitoral engorgement are important precursors of orgasm in women, and Viagra may help women who have difficulty reaching orgasm as well.

Though it may seem hard to believe, the story of Viagra for women may be even bigger than the men's stampede we've just witnessed.

As a female psychiatrist, my perspective on erectile dysfunction and Viagra in men and women is a unique one. In the conclusion, I'll discuss how Viagra will affect relationships and living and loving in the next century. A new sexual revolution is upon us, a medical advance that can make the length of our sexual life more closely approximate our life span. What really matters in the end is less the drug itself than the people who take it, less the details of the problem than how individuals and couples handle it. It may sound corny to some and self-evident to others, but Viagra really does raise issues that are at the heart of our views of men, women, and couples.

Viagra will force us to confront our values about what matters in relationships and challenge our beliefs about love, intimacy, and mortality. As Shakespeare said, it's a brave new world that has such creatures in it.

The problem of impotence is an age-old problem. It seemed like the ultimate punishment as far back as Genesis, when God smote Abimelech with its scourge in response to Abimelech's adulterous thoughts about Abraham's wife, Sarah. By the time Cleopatra's face had launched a thousand ships, men were making offerings to idols in ancient Egypt in hopes that the gods of fate would make their masts rise as well. Across the way in Greece, men were drinking potions concocted from the blood of gelded rams while a young Iphiclus—foreshadowing Freud's Oedipus—became impotent after his father came too close for comfort, showing his son one of the knives used in the gelding process. In a maneuver Freud would have appreciated, a kindly physician then restored Iphiclus to psychological (and sexual) health by helping him master his fear of his father's knife. A new (and somewhat unfortunate) psychology of impotence was born.

The witchcraft, hexes, and spells of the Dark Ages gradually gave way to the Enlightenment, the Age of Reason. If it looks like a penis, some speculated, eating it may help mine. Diets of carrots, cucumbers, and bananas—not to mention rhinoceros horn (high in calcium and very crunchy)—became very popular in Europe. Animal parts, especially the testicles of large animals, were popular accompaniments, perhaps on the theory that anyone who would eat them must have balls. Oysters, those tasty testicles of the sea, were popped like penile Prozac as well. It was the Age of Reason, but it dawned slowly.

By the sixteenth century, physicians got interested in sex for the first time when Varolio, an Italian physician, noted that blood flowed through the penis. Understanding how the body worked was the project of the day, and even Michelangelo dissected and drew the male member. The result? The famously flaccid but well-endowed David. Leonardo (the pre-DiCaprio one) also had a strong interest in the mechanics of sexual functioning.

Casual chemists for centuries concocted potions in their caves and kitchens to assist them in their lovemaking, often stumbling on remedies that contained substances currently available only by prescription today. For example, the jimsonweed used in America and the mandrake popular in Eurasia are both members of the nightshade plant family. These nightshades, related to the deadly nightshade plant known as belladonna, contain alkaloids such as those found in morphine that appear to affect the part of the brain that triggers erections as well as reducing the effects of adrenaline on the penis. Since you don't want an erection at a moment where you must fight or flee, adrenaline (and the anxiety that produces it) are anathema for erections.

Ultimately, though, it was the ever-popular poppy plant that produced the papaverine that set in motion the modern research that culminated in Viagra. In the shot felt round the world, French surgeon Ronald Virag reported that during surgery, he had accidentally injected the nitrogen-containing compound into the corpus cavernosum, the wrong part of his patient's penis. The anesthetized patient spiked a two-hour erection while out like a light, to the chagrin and then the intrigue of the entire surgical team, giving nocturnal erections new meaning.

It took nearly two decades longer to find an oral solution to the impotence problem, potency in pill form. Meanwhile men winced while injecting themselves in the penis or inserting tiny pills in the urethra. Unlike Viagra, which requires erotic psychological involvement as well as physical penile stimulation to work, these earlier treatments were impersonal and unwieldy, the effects of medication on man rather than man on medication. A sudden flat tire, the wife's unheralded headache, or a date's change of heart and you've still got that erection for hours, a penis with a will of its own, no room for the wishes of the man attached. It was hard to blame the women for their sense that the erection was impersonal and mechanical.

Now, eighteen years after that fateful first injection, the new revolution of sexual medicine is upon us, and you can be part of it.

Viagra.

Even its name seems meant to evoke the thundering power of Niagara Falls, that gushing cascade of natural beauty central to so many honeymoons. The force behind the stampede to get it is precisely about honeymoons—the chance to have those second sexual honeymoons that seemed lost forever to aging or disease. The discovery of Viagra, simply put, is in many ways as exciting and valuable as the discovery of the mythical Fountain of Youth.

Viagra's journey to stardom began in a lab, where it was a humdrum cardiovascular drug that was failing its tests. It didn't help with angina (the chest pain usually produced by atherosclerosis, the blockage of the coronary arteries with fatty deposits), but for some reason, at the end of the clinical trials, the patients were reluctant to give it back.

Researchers soon learned that Viagra wasn't making blood rush to cardiac patients' hearts, but it was indeed making it rush to another organ. Recognizing serendipity when they saw it, the reseachers shifted gears. They quickly found that Viagra caused smooth muscle dilation in the arteries that allowed increased blood flow in penile tissue, amplifying the usual cascade of cellular events that produce the blood engorgement that leads to erections. At one test site, the locked box in which the Viagra that the researchers were testing was being stored was raided in the middle of the night. Researchers returned the next morning to find the lock broken and the Viagra gone. In contrast, the heavy-duty, controlled-substance pain medications sitting right beside the Viagra—narcotics worth a fortune on the street—were left untouched. Wow, the researchers realized. This stuff is good. It was a sign of things to come.

With Viagra, the gauntlet has been thrown. Can you and your partner enjoy a lifetime of excellent, satisfying sex? Are you willing to do what it takes, even if that means more than just popping a pill?

How could a sexual revolution revolve around a pill? Although we'd like to think that past shifts hinged on changes of heart and mind—for instance, the sudden realization that Victorian piano legs weren't really so sexually provocative after all—the truth is that sexual shifts are more frequently the result of technology: the invention of rubber(s), the birth control pill. Each of these advances pushed sex in a new direction. Viagra will, too. When it works, it means that now you can have sex when, where, and how you want it, dependably and reliably, even if you're one hundred and your partner's one hundred and two. If it's true that every revolution needs a theme song, the Age of Viagra's may be hip-hop artist George Clinton's "Hard as Steel." Clinton observes that "play-dough" dough boys are out and "hard-as-steel" stud muffins are in. What will having the "fantasy penis" really mean for men, women, and sex? Stay tuned.

Among the questions of the day are:

- Does Viagra represent the beginning of our recognition of a new midlife change for men, a menopausal equivalent that Gail Sheehy has dubbed "man-o-pause"?
- What will it teach us about so-called normal aging in men? Could it do for men what hormone replacement therapy has done for women's sexuality in midlife?
- What about reports that Viagra, taken regularly, can actually prevent the onset of erectile dysfunction the way hormone replacement therapy prevents osteoporosis in women?

What of the effects of Viagra on male sexuality more generally? Will potency in pill form mean that men who once hammed it up in the locker room, bragging about their conquests, will be a thing of the past? After all, if anyone can buy the pill, anyone can be a sexual superstud.

Will Viagra mean that the psychological meaning attached to erections ebbs, since now anyone can get them by popping a pill? Or will the new male line be, "Hey, baby, I'm a natural. No Viagra in these veins." Surely women will be just as impressed as they have been by past male pick-up lines. But if men whose steps have lost their spring are suddenly hot to trot, who will they want to trot with? Their wives or some new spring chicken from the office?

Then there's the Prozac Problem. Is Viagra merely another instance of cosmetic psychopharmacology, neurochemical buffing in the absence of any real disorder, a kind of Wonderbra for men trying to defy the effects of gravity and aging? Will men end up taking pills to fix what's not broken? Or will the fact that the pills help redefine what "broken" means the way that Prozac redefined "depression"? Is it all right to take a pill to be better than normal? And does that make it a medication or a recreational drug?

Finally, what of the insurance question? Will the companies pay for Viagra as if it were any other medicine, like insulin or antibiotics? How many pills constitutes a one-month supply? Two a day? Two a week? Two a month? Who will decide how many erections are enough? How will managed care manage Viagra?

As a psychiatrist, I have long been interested in questions of mind and brain. Psychiatry has been notoriously disdainful of cures that involve external solutions rather than internal ones, say a trip abroad to cure depression instead of good, old-fashioned introspection. As a psychoanalyst by training, I have also been a proponent of psychotherapy, of changing your mind through the slow, laborious process of changing your brain, neuron by neuron. My first book, *The Talking Cure: The Science Behind Psychotherapy,* was an attempt to synthesize a new understanding of how psychotherapy works to effect permanent brain changes.

Now we have a pill that can produce an overnight shift in the sexual functioning of men that may have been impaired for years. What will that mean for relationships? With Viagra, the stage is set for the biggest social experiment of our time, an unusual opportunity to explore the interface of the physical, the psychological, and the sexual. If there's one thing psychoanalysts know well, it's that sexuality is central to our existence, our core identities, and our happiness. It's fundamentally intertwined with who we are, how we feel. As the old analytic joke goes, "Everything is about sex except sex, which is about aggression." But I'm betting that sex is about sex, too. There are more questions than answers, but one thing is clear—this is an exciting time.

If you've ever stood by Niagara Falls and felt the

energy, the electricity in the air, you're prepared for the sensation that is Viagra. Every man will have his own metaphor for Viagra's effects, from feeling turbocharged to getting his roar back, from feeling bullish on the future to being ready to play hardball. Regaining erectile strength and power will inevitably affect a man's sense of who he is as a man.

As Ted put it after his first dose, "Before Viagra, I felt I'd been put out to pasture, sexually speaking. But now I feel like a cowboy again, maybe even the Marlboro Man. Minus the cigarettes, of course. But packing something even better instead. Now Sarah and I can ride off into our sunset years together as a team."

Are you ready to get back up in the saddle and ride like you were eighteen again? Read on.

PART 1

The Impotence
Problem

1

The Plumbing and Circuitry
of the Penis

This chapter is a penile primer, an owner's manual to the manly organ. Even an Erector set comes with instructions, but a penis comes with none. Like most men, you'll probably recall that your parents didn't exactly fill you in on the inner workings of your private parts. Chances are that the closest you got to a tour of that subterranean world below the belt was high school biology. So in this chapter I'll give you an overview of the equipment involved in erections, the fuel lines that turbocharge the penis and the electrical circuitry that drives them. You're probably more comfortable with your auto mechanic when you understand what he thinks is wrong with your car and what he's proposing to do about it. When you know a carburetor from a generator, chances are you'll get a better repair job. The same is true when you speak to your internist, urologist, or psychiatrist about Viagra. What follows is a discussion from your penis's perspective, a chance for you to learn how erections work from the inside out.

NOT ONE ROD, BUT THREE

"Rod," the street slang used to refer to the penis, is correct in one sense but wrong in another. Actually, the penis is three rods, one underneath and two sitting side by side on top of it. The penis triples your pleasure with three rods in one. But let's call these rods by their technical names. The flexible rod on the underside of the penis is called the corpus spongiosum, literally meaning "spongy body," because it is indeed made from a spongelike tissue. It begins at the base of the penis and ends at the tip of the penis with the glans penis, the "head." The urethra, a tube that carries urine from the bladder as well as semen from the testes, runs smack through the middle of the corpus spongiosum, ending at the tip of the glans. Between the bladder and the penis, the urethra is surrounded by the prostate gland, which forms a ring around the urethra that can all too easily become a cuff that constricts it. True to its name, the corpus spongiosum remains spongy even during erections. The dual importance of its sponginess will become clear momentarily.

Lying atop the corpus spongiosum, the spongy rod containing the urethra, are two chambers that power the penis like the double barrels of a shotgun. These chambers are called the corpus cavernosum, or "cavernous bodies," because—like seaside caves that fill with water when the tide comes in—they fill with blood when sexual excitement mounts. The corpus cavernosum is actually made up of sponge-like tissue with millions of tiny pockets that are usually empty and flat. What keeps the pockets empty is the constant work of the smooth muscle cells that are liberally scattered throughout the corpus cavernosum. These cells limit the flow of traffic of blood into the penis by clamping down the way a reluctant drawbridge operator with his bridge clamped shut blocks boat traffic. Without the constant ironclad grip of these smooth muscle cells, men would walk around with erections all the time. But when the reticent drawbridge operator loosens up, boats can pass freely into port. Similarly, when the uptight smooth muscle cells relax, blood can move into the penis, expanding the normally empty pockets of the corpus cavernosum up to sixfold. That movement of blood is what causes an erection. Think of water balloons that go from limp to filled.

But unlike elastic balloons, the outer covering of the corpus cavernosum, known as the tunica albuginea (a term designed to bug medical students) is stiff and inflexible, more like a sheath rather than a flowing tunic. This inelasticity means two main things: First, when blood flows into the penis, it expands a lot, but like your stomach, there are limits to how much it can expand. The tunica serves as a straightjacket of sorts, forming an impromptu container that can withstand the pressure of the penis filling with blood. The stiff wall serves another equally important function as well. You may remember from Biology 101 that arteries are the blood vessels that carry blood from the heart to the organs, where it courses through tiny capillaries before returning to the heart through the veins. Where the arteries are tough and muscular, not easily squeezed, the veins are flabby and lax, as easy to collapse as a garden hose under the foot of a large man. The veins that drain blood from the penis get pressed upon by the growing pressure of the blood that surrounds them in the corpus cavernosum. They collapse, trapping blood in the penis the way a drain stopper traps water in a tub. So the tunica albuginea guarantees that when blood checks into the penis, it won't check out—at least not for the half hour or so that the job at hand requires.

By now the wisdom of God's decision to put the urethra in the corpus spongiosum may be becoming clear to you, since if the urethra ran through tissue that tumesced rather than sponged during erections, it would be clamped shut like a garden hose, too. If that were to happen, all those billions and billions of sperm couldn't swim upstream to spawn. Furthermore, if the corpus spongiosum were as hard as each corpus cavernosum is when erect, women would scream in pain every time the glans penis pummeled their cervix during intercourse.

Now that you know where the cylinders and exhaust pipes are, let's take a look at the fuel lines and the electrical wiring that make the penis roar. The fuel lines that supply the gasoline to spark erections are the penile arteries, one to each corpus cavernosum. Very straightforward, they are branches of branches of branches of branches of the aorta. A deep cavernosal artery brings blood to each corpus cavernosum, taking it from flaccidity to tumescence to rigidity. A deep cavernosal vein drains the blood away from each corpus cavernosum as the erection wanes. If turbocharging our cars were this simple, they'd spend far less time in the shop. As we'll see in the next chapter, these seemingly straightforward fuel lines that power the penis can certainly cause a lot of trouble. Blockages of these amorous arteries, each the size of one tine of a fork, are most often responsible for gumming up the works, sexually speaking.

POINT AND SHOOT

The neuron-based electrical wiring responsible for pointing and shooting (erection and ejaculation) is a bit more complicated. It's worth understanding, because it may help you map out the potential causes of nerve-related potency problems.

Like other organs, the penis is essentially controlled by the autonomic nervous system, which might be thought of as the automatic nervous system: It's responsible for all involuntary motor activities, such as erections. The voluntary or somatic nervous system also innervates the penis: The sensory branch tells you when the penile skin is stroked and the motor branch tenses the pelvic muscles that surround the penis's base. As most men with impotence know, erections are beyond conscious control and the penis isn't a muscle to be tensed. All the willing and wishing, all the huffing and puffing in the world won't help if it isn't doing it involuntarily. Heavy petting with a special pet may send a signal up the wiring from your penis to your brain to fill it in on what's going on down under, but it's your autonomic nervous system that will determine whether your pet gets a rise out of you. When the penis is stimulated, it either goes on autopilot or it doesn't.

The autonomic nervous system is in turn broken down into two equal and opposing parts, the parasympathetic nervous system and the sympathetic nervous system. Despite their lengthy names, these two systems are well known to you: The parasympathetic system is the one at play when you are relaxed, say digesting a big meal while vegging out on the couch watching television or drinking that glass of wine by the fire with your beloved, anticipating the evening's erotic activities. This parasympathetic system depends on a neurotransmitter, a conduction chemical, known as acetylcholine. Hold that thought.

The sympathetic nervous system, in contrast, is

the one that operates when you're ready to fight or flee. It relies on adrenaline to speed its messages along from nerve to nerve, like a petrified Pony Express rider who has just seen a stagecoach robbery in progress and narrowly escapes with his life.

Which brings us to point and shoot, erection and ejaculation. Erection, the process of pointing your penis like a bird dog indicating prey, depends on the parasympathetic nervous system. Ejaculation, the process of shooting, relies on the sympathetic nervous system. So for sex to go well for men, they have to be able to both point and shoot. Simply put, both parts of your nervous system must be working well in order for you to point and shoot. Right away you can probably see why anxiety—a kind of misguided desire to fight or flee in response to an internally generated sense of impending doom—is anathema to erectile functioning. To point, you have to be in relaxation mode. To shoot, you go into the other mode.

Erection = parasympathetic activity = relaxation

Ejaculation = sympathetic activity = fight-or-flee

INSIDE THE CYLINDERS

So now that we've peeked into your penis the way you might look under the hood of your car to see the parts that make it tick, let's watch it in action. To really understand how a car runs, you need to peer inside the carburetor and watch as the pounding cylinders trigger tiny explosion after explosion, injecting just enough gasoline to keep the whole thing running. That kind of up-close inspection of the corpus cavernosum during erections will help you understand what makes your penis purr—and what makes Viagra work.

The true fuel that makes the corpus cavernosum tick is nitric oxide. If we could zoom inside your caverns like a spelunker with a searchlight to watch what makes the blood start to engorge the penis in the first place, what we'd find is the following: In response to hearing from the nerves that they're turned on, the endothelial cells that line the corpus cavernosum, which already have some nitric oxide hanging around, start to manufacture more in a manic manner. The increase in nitric oxide triggers a remarkable and coordinated effort reminiscent of those men passing sandbags down a line so as to save a town from a raging river. Only this time the goal is not to dam up the river but to flood the penis. And as each sandbag is passed along, it energizes the others. As more sandbags are passed along, the whole chain works faster and other chemicals are produced: guanylate cyclase and cGMP (cyclic guanosine

monophosphate), a powerhouse that can ̇
the most uptight of smooth muscle cells relȧ
chemicals make the cells let their guard dȯ
blood flows into the penis. The once-wilted ̇and
becomes magically erect and the Love Boat sets sail.

However, there's a culprit below deck, a Love
Boat saboteur known as the mysterious enzyme
PDE5. PDE5 is phosphodiesterase type 5, whose
dastardly deed is to erode the strength of cGMP.
You remember cGMP, our tall, dark, and handsome
powerhouse whose job it is to loosen up the smooth
muscle cells that keep the Love Boat tied to the pier.
The villainous enzyme PDE5 drains cGMP's energy, in effect tying one hand behind his back. PDE5
slows cGMP's efforts to relax the smooth muscle
cells and produce the blood flood that is erection. By
gradually breaking down our hero, PDE5 in effect
tightens the reins on the corpus cavernosum. Like a
too-short vacation that's over before it's even begun,
the Love Boat is on its way to losing steam even as
it's just leaving port.

That happens even in the normal penis.

**cGMP makes smooth muscle cells
relax so that blood enters the penis**

PDE5 breaks down cGMP

Viagra counteracts PDE5

Enter Viagra, to save the day. Viagra works by taking on the villain, PDE5. It keeps PDE5 from degrading our powerhouse cGMP. With more cGMP around, the smooth muscle cells in the corpus cavernosum are more relaxed. Once again, the Love Boat can set sail.

That's why with Viagra on board men feel like they're eighteen again, when a whiff of perfume could still make them stiff for hours. You can understand why Viagra is helpful for a wide range of erectile problems, whether they stem from arterial damage, nerve damage, or psychological factors. Even if a man is only able to get a little nitric oxide going, Viagra can boost that natural response, magnify and make more of it simply by blocking the effects of PDE5. In that way, Viagra's not really doing anything artificial, just tilting the balance in nitric oxide's favor, doing what comes naturally, and accentuating the positive.

Like any pill, Viagra does have side effects, ranging from headaches to an upset stomach to changes in your blue-green color vision. The details of these will be explored in depth in Chapter 6. As we'll see later, all these strange side effects arise from Viagra's inhibition of various subtypes of PDE in other parts of the body. Because it's an oral medication, when you swallow this Mighty Mouse of a pill, it doesn't just go to your groin but circulates throughout your whole body.

Relatively minor side effects aside, perhaps the

biggest unexpected psychological effect of Viagra is that men simply feel younger. Beware. But it's quite possible to keep all the wisdom contained in the brain of a sixty-five-year-old man intact, even if his penis acts like a kid again. That may make for the best sex of all. A little spring fever never hurt anyone.

2

The Physical Causes
of Impotence

If you're reading a book on Viagra, it's likely that
your Love Boat has felt more like the *Titanic* on
more than one occasion. This chapter will show you
where you hit an iceberg and how to make it to a
lifeboat, sexually speaking. Viagra may make men
(and perhaps even their doctors) gloss over the
reasons for their difficulties. After all, it seems to be
a cure that tends to work whatever the cause of the
impotence. But erectile dysfunction (ED) can be
caused by many things that you need to know about,
not mask. Things that can affect your overall physical health, such as atherosclerosis (clogging of the
arteries caused by high levels of cholesterol) and
diabetes mellitus, which can damage your penis's
electrical wiring as well as its arterial fuel lines. It's
important to know you have atherosclerosis before a
heart attack, given that only 50% of men survive

their first one. A quarter of men with erectile dysfunction have a heart attack or stroke in the two years after their penile problems present. It's also important to learn of diabetes before your vision is damaged beyond repair. Erectile dysfunction is often the very first sign of diabetes. The causes of impotence are many, and ultimately they all flow from problems with the arterial fuel lines and electrical circuitry examined in the last chapter.

What's Gunking Up Those Fuel Lines?

Simply put, the main fuel line problem that the penis is prone to is blockage of its arteries, those fork-tine-thin fuel lines that provide blood power to the phallus. Generally speaking, it's what you've put *on* your fork tines all those years that causes the problem: that weekly steak, the accompanying potato with sour cream and butter, the chocolate mousse that topped it off. The process of blockage of the arteries begins at a surprisingly young age, in men in their early twenties. So whether the problem rears its ugly head at forty or seventy, chances are it's actually been evolving for years. Erectile dysfunction occurs in 40% of men at age forty and 70% of men at age seventy. The trouble may not strike until you're paying college tuition bills for your children, but it often dates back to your own college days of double-decker bacon cheeseburgers at the drive-in.

The risk factors for arterial blockage of the penile arteries are the same as those for blockage of the coronary arteries that supply the heart. Smoking, obesity, high cholesterol, high blood pressure, and diabetes are the primary modifiable culprits, though family history and genetics also play a role. Not surprisingly, these so-called lifestyle factors are all intertwined. Obesity is a result of the overeating of fatty foods that are high in cholesterol and saturated fats, foods that raise serum cholesterol and triglyceride levels. Obesity also causes an increased chance of diabetes, because the overly plump fat cells of overly plump people are less responsive to insulin than they should be. In addition, obesity helps encourage a sedentary lifestyle that makes it difficult to lose weight and control diabetes. Finally, obesity is linked to high blood pressure, which in effect pounds away at the arteries, damaging their delicate inner lining and leaving them ripe for deposits of cholesterol to form.

So the puffy couch potato watching TV while smoking and eating Fritos is a setup for diabetes, high blood pressure, and high serum cholesterol, while having a slim chance of controlling it. In contrast, his athletic roommate who eats right and exercises is less likely to get diabetes or hypertension or high serum cholesterol, because he isn't fat. That is why his penis, like his belly, is probably rock hard at fifty while his couch potato friend's belly and penis are both flabby and flaccid. The couch potato's love handles mean that he can't handle lovemaking as well anymore, as great a guy as he may be otherwise. So if your belt seems to be getting shorter as your belly expands, you're setting yourself up for problems below the belt as well. So the next time you spear a big hunk of red meat with your fork, remember your fork-tine-thin fuel lines and think again.

You may have read somewhere that a large glass of red wine that accompanies a steak will wash away the fat, keeping your arteries squeaky clean. In fact, alcohol in moderation (no more than a drink a day) does in fact reduce your risk of the atherosclerotic disease that can clog your coronary and penile arteries. But if you have diabetes, watch out, because even moderate amounts of alcohol in diabetics make the vascular disease it produces worse. Although alcohol may assist you in terms of atherosclerosis, taken chronically in even moderate excess, it has well-documented negative effects on both testosterone levels and libido. So at best, that martini is a mixed blessing. It may help keep your fuel lines open if you don't have diabetes, but taken to excess it actually reduces desire.

Many people also think that lack of exercise is a risk factor when it comes to atherosclerosis, but this is probably true only indirectly. Exercise helps people control their weight (which in turn reduces the risk of diabetes), blood pressure, and cholesterol levels. Since sex is a physical sport of sorts, the better shape you're in, the more likely you are to enjoy yourself without pulling something or panting for breath. Feeling lean and mean often means that your self-esteem, a powerful determinant of how psychologically footloose and fancy free you feel, will be pumped up as well.

Having a Type A (Aggressive/Ambitious) personality is a problem only if it leads to smoking, overeating, elevated cholesterol, and a sedentary lifestyle that promotes obesity and ultimately diabetes and hypertension. It is not, however, a direct risk factor in and of itself. So if you can channel your aggressive ambitiousness into remaining fit and trim, being a Type A type won't necessarily hurt you, at least not atherosclerotically speaking.

Now let's look at what happens to those smooth muscle cells responsible for clamping down and keeping blood out of your penis most of the time. As the penile arteries gradually narrow due to more and more gunky ghosts of cholesterol past, the smooth muscle cells literally starve to death for oxygen while mired in the muck. They are transformed into fibrocytes, which, as the name suggests, are fibrous cells (similar to those found in scars) that are much more rigid, much more difficult to loosen up than the smooth muscle cells they replace. The corpus cavernosum loses its expansiveness and elasticity. Blood has a harder time getting in, and erectile function suffers accordingly.

It's worth eliminating the risk factors for atherosclerosis before it's a problem, a goal that is mainly accomplished through diet and exercise. Once you have atherosclerosis you'll probably develop impotence (not to mention the risk of having a heart attack or a stroke), and if you're put on a medication such as an antihypertensive to reduce your risk factors, you may have problems from side effects. Suffice it to say that atherosclerotic risk factors and many of the drugs used to treat them are a Catch-22. It's better to catch atherosclerosis when *you're* twenty-two. Remember what they say about an ounce of prevention: It's worth a pound of Viagra.

Trauma to the pelvic area can also produce injuries to the crucial penile arteries, usually by causing shearing that damages them in one location. But problems with the veins that drain the penis of blood when your erection wanes are very rare. It's really the amorous arteries that reduce the fuel to your tool when blocked. If you can't get hard, you can't compress the veins that drain the penis within the corpus cavernosum. With this problem, known as veno-occlusive dysfunction, the vein is not occluded or flattened, because there is not a high enough amount of pressure in the corpus cavernosum to flatten it. Instead of that large man who stepped on the garden hose, picture a little child standing on it instead. Water can still flow through. When the blood isn't trapped, the penis is like a bathtub with the stopper left out of the drain: blood may be flowing in, but the overall level doesn't rise, because water is draining almost as fast as it's coming in. Erectile dysfunction, once present, in effect makes itself worse by failing to exert enough pressure to occlude the veins.

The medications used to treat the risk factors for atherosclerosis, such as hypertension, can generally be thought of as cardiovascular killjoys. Many of them cause potency problems, monkeying around with the arterial supply throughout the body, including affecting the penis. These drugs are heartless, knowing that you can't live without them and making it difficult for you to live with them, too.

The medications most likely to affect potency are listed below and on subsequent pages. You probably know them best by their brand names, which appear in parentheses.

Central sympathomimetics, which are activators of the sympathetic nervous system, are anything but sympathetic to your erectile efforts:

- Clonadine (Catapress, Combipres)
- Methyldopa (Aldomet, Aldoclor, Aldoril)
- Reserpine (Diupres, Metatensin, Regroton, Salutensin, Serpasil)
- Rauwolfia serpentina (Harmonyl, Raudixin, Rauside)

I've always thought rauwolfia sounded like a raw wolf with fangs like a serpent. He'll take a bite out of your erectile function if you let him.

Beta-blockers, which reduce the heart's workload and relax the arteries, are used for everything from coronary artery disease to high blood pressure. Easy to recognize because they all end in -olol:

- Timolol (Blocadren, Timolide, Timoptic)
- Propranolol (Inderal, Inderide, Inderide LA)
- Metoprolol (Lopressor, Lopressor HCT, Toprol-XL)
- Atenolol (Tenormin, Tenoretic)
- Bisoprolol (Zebeta, Ziac)
- Sotalol (Betapace)
- Esmolol (Brevibloc)
- Carteolol (Cartrol)
- Betaxolol (Kerlone, Betoptic)
- Penbutolol (Levatol)
- Acebutolol (Sectral)

Diuretics reduce the overall blood volume by getting the kidney to kick out more salt and water from the body. This lowers the blood pressure and leaves you heading for the bathroom day and night. Diuretics are likely to make you piss away your phallic power:

- Spironolactone (Aldactazide, Aldactone)
- Hydrochlorthiazide (Aldactazide, Apresazide, Dyazide, Esidris, HydroDIURIL, Hydropres, Moduretic, Ser-Ap-Es, Maxzide, Microzide)
- Chlorthiazide (Diuril)
- Chlorthalidone (Demi-regroton, Hygroton, Oretic)
- Amiloride (Midamor)

Other bad guys that are unwanted in bed include:

- Clofibrate (Atromid-S) and Gemfibrizol (Lopid), both medications to control high cholesterol
- Digitalis (Crystodigin, Lanoxicaps, Lanoxin), a medication that improves cardiac function and blocks arrhythmias
- Phenoxybenzamine (Dibenzyline), an antihypertensive that blocks alpha rather than beta receptors
- Disopyramide (Norpace), a medication for arrhythmias
- Guanethidine (Esimil, Ismelin), which blocks responses to the sympathetic nervous system

Luckily for you and your lover, there are also some good guys around who can help your hypertension without increasing marital tension. For instance, ACE Inhibitors probably fight hypertension by inhibiting angiotensin-converting enzyme (ACE). Because this enzyme needed for blood vessel constriction is blocked, the vessels relax instead. The following medications are your ACE in the hole when it comes to hypertensive cures that aren't heartless to your love life (all with the suffix -pril):

- Quinapril (Accupril)
- Enalapril (Vasotec)
- Benzapril (Lotensin)
- Captopril (Catopen)
- Fosinopril (Monopril)

- Lisinopril (Zestrin)
- Ramipril (Altace)

Other good guys include:

- Amlodipine (Norvasc) and Nifedipine (Procardia), calcium-channel blockers that can effectively lower your blood pressure
- Prazosin (Minipress), a antihypertensive with an incidence of impotence under 1%

Arterial Fuel Line Problems

1. Atherosclerosis produced by risk factors including:
   - Smoking
   - Obesity
   - High Cholesterol
   - Hypertension (high blood pressure)
   - Diabetes
2. Diabetes
3. Cardiovascular Medications
4. Trauma or Surgery

ELECTRICAL SHORTS

As we learned earlier, the penis's wiring consists of complicated circuitry, neurologically speaking. Electrical shorts anywhere in the system can lead to the interruption of the impulses that produce penile potency. These nerves may have blown a fuse. They may have been damaged for a wide range of reasons. But the problem with these blown circuits is that they can't be turned on again like a circuit breaker that's been tripped.

Remember that erection and ejaculation, pointing and shooting, are controlled by the parasympathetic and sympathetic nervous systems. Each of these systems has parts that originate in the brain and spinal cord and course through the spinal cord before forming spiderweblike networks of nerves that ultimately end up in the pudendal nerve of the penis. Since the wiring diagram for the penis runs from the brain down the spinal cord and out from the spinal cord to the penis itself, there are plenty of opportunities for problems due to interruption of service at each level. Let's look at the levels one by one.

"IT'S ALL IN YOUR HEAD"

This unfortunate statement, to which many impotent men have been subjected over time, has some limited merit. There are psychological reasons for impotence that we will discuss in more detail in the next chapter. In general, these include negative emotions toward sex such as anxiety, guilt, anger, or disgust. Negative emotions can produce a so-called adrenergic response, which means that the sympathetic nervous system, which uses noradrenaline at its synapses (the junctions between nerve cells), is overly active. You'll recall that such sympathetic outflow is anything but sympathetic to your erection. Lack of desire, which can be caused by either psychological or physical factors, can also be an "all in your head" reason for erectile dysfunction. Although we will discuss psychological reasons for impotence in more detail in the next chapter, it is crucially important to note that all mind problems are in fact ultimately problems of the brain. Your thoughts, feelings, and fantasies, which arise within the brain, hook up with your point-and-shoot apparatus in important ways, usually by causing anxiety or through lack of desire. Erection depends on relaxation, which is the predominance of cholinergic rather than adrenergic tone within the autonomic nervous system. Anxiety arising from psychological conflicts can tip this balance in favor of the fight-or-flight sympathetic system that makes erection impossible. The brain is also in charge of desire, so alterations in this first step of the sexual response cycle can also lead to problems with erectile functioning.

Many nonpsychiatrists note that we are increasingly learning that impotence is a problem with physiological rather than psychological causes. As a psychiatrist, however, I would argue that *all* causes of impotence, including the so-called psychological ones, are ultimately physiological. The real question is whether the cause will affect the way the problem is treated medically. Since there's good reason to think that Viagra will treat erectile dysfunction arising from a wide range of causes, making this distinction may be less important than it sounds like it would be. To me, anything that makes it clear that the brain is the organ of the mind and that mind problems are ultimately brain problems is good for psychiatric patients, whose stigmatization is often based on the notion that their problems are not real because they are "all in their heads."

Other brain problems besides a preponderance of anxiety or a lack of desire can cause erectile dysfunction as well. For example, Parkinson's disease results from the dying off of some neurons in the brain responsible for movement. Parkinson's can lead to erectile dysfunction because the brain cells that die are linked to the parasympathetic part of the autonomic nervous system. Drugs used to treat Parkinson's disease can also wreak havoc on erectile functioning by affecting the operation of important nerves:

- Trihexyphenidyl (Artane)
- Benztropine (Cogentin)
- Procyclidine (Kemadrin)

Multiple sclerosis, a disease in which nerve cells lose their protective, insulating outer myelin sheaths, can lead to erectile dysfunction by affecting nerves that are part of the autonomic nervous system in either the brain or the spinal cord. In effect, these nerves look like stereo speaker wire that has been punctured by staples as you tried to tack it to the wall. Like that punctured wire, these nerves don't play right.

STRIKING THE WRONG CORD

The spinal cord is a relay station for the autonomic nervous system where connections are made between nerve cells. Anything that disrupts the flow of electrical impulses along the spinal cord can cause erectile problems as well. Although the spinal cord is protected by the bony vertebrae that make up your backbone, serious injuries such as those arising from car, bicycle, motorcycle, and diving accidents can sever the cord, causing a disconnection of the penile circuitry from the brain. This disconnection can also be caused by cancers of the spinal cord, strokes involving the spinal cord, and other illnesses that disrupt the wiring along the way. If the cord is struck in the wrong way, erectile dysfunction is the result. Because the sympathetic nervous system travels this route as well, problems with orgasm and ejaculation can also occur.

THE PHALLIC PERIPHERY

Once the parasympathetic and sympathetic nerves leave the spinal cord, they form networks of neurons that ultimately end up at their destination, the penis.

These so-called peripheral nerves—peripheral to your brain and spinal cord, but certainly not to your phallic pleasure —can develop many different types of problems that mess up the wiring.

The most common problem in this part of this circuitry is diabetes mellitus, a disorder in which the pancreas fails to produce enough insulin to regulate the level of sugar (glucose) in your blood stream. Different from the diabetes some people develop in childhood or adolescence (Juvenile onset, or Type I diabetes, which is hereditary and requires insulin injections), most diabetes is acquired in adult life by people whose overstuffed fat cells are less responsive to insulin than they would be if they were smaller. Diabetes causes leaky cell membranes in nerves that ultimately cause structural damage to the wiring itself, in addition to providing the previously discussed risk factor for atherosclerosis. Recent estimates suggest that between 35 and 75% of men with diabetes mellitus face erectile dysfunction. The risk of this complication goes up as patients have diabetes for longer and longer periods of time. So diabetes causes a double whammy, affecting both your fuel lines and your electrical wiring simultaneously.

Likewise, any surgical or other traumatic damage to the penile nerves can produce erectile dysfunction. These causes may range from a too-hard bike seat that causes nerve compression to damage to the pelvis in an accident. In short, they are largely the same ones responsible for arterial damage through trauma. Some damage is actually doctor-induced, caused by prostate surgery or other pelvic or lower gastrointestinal surgeries such as those for colorectal and bladder cancers that disrupt the pudendal nerves.

Prostate cancer affects some 300,000 American men annually, and you may recall from the previous chapter that the prostate wraps around the urethra between the bladder and the base of the penis. So surgery to remove a prostate riddled with cancer takes place very near to the penis and its all-important, potency-producing nerves. A radical prostatectomy, in which the prostate is removed due to cancer, often results in a great deal of nerve damage even when so-called nerve-sparing surgery is done. Other options, like the implantation of tiny radioactive pellets directly into the prostate gland, can also cause nerve damage that results in varying degrees of erectile dysfunction. While Viagra success rates are somewhat lower for prostate cancer survivors than others with impotence, the drug can help many of them as well.

Medications that are used to treat what we think of as psychiatric or neurological disorders are also prime producers of potency problems. A simple way to think of them is that they generally work on psychiatric illnesses such as depression and anxiety by affecting nerve cells in the brain, but they also affect nerve cells in the rest of the body as well. These medications affect the way the nerves operate, often shifting the precarious balance between the sympathetic and parasympathetic nervous system tone that is so important in erection and ejaculation. Many psychotropic medications (that is, those that change your psyche and brain) can affect your erectile function and sexual performance.

Antidepressants: The antidepressants that cause impotence read like a who's who of psychiatric medication.

Tricyclics may elevate your mood, but you may be depressed to see their effects on your penis:

- Clomipramine (Anafranil)
- Nortriptyline (Aventyl, Pamelor)
- Desipramine (Norpramin, Pertofrane)
- Imipramine (Janimine, Tofranil)
- Amitriptyline (Elavil, Etrafon, Endep)
- Trimipramine (Surmontil)
- Protriptyline (Vivactil)

MAO Inhibitors mean people can't enjoy the red wine and cheese appetizers that so often precede sexual play, because they block your ability to digest tyramine, an amino acid found in protein, and too much tyramine can cause your blood pressure to skyrocket:

- Tranylcypromatine (Parnate)
- Phenylzine (Nardil)

Selective serotonin reuptake inhibitors (SSRIs), the class of which Prozac is king, can reduce your ability to get and keep an erection. Even worse, they can also reduce your libido and increase the amount of time it takes to reach orgasm or even completely prevent you from reaching it:

- Fluoxetine (Prozac)
- Sertraline (Zoloft)
- Paroxetine (Paxil)

Antidepressants that will make you happy in bed as well include:

- Fluvoxamine (Luvox), which stands alone among the SSRIs in not producing sexual dysfunction
- Nefazodone (Serzone)
- Venlafaxine (Effexor)
- Buproprion (Wellbutrin)

Mood stabilizers and anticonvulsants that can be problematic include:

- Lithium (Eskalith, Lithan, Lithobid, Lithonate, Lithotabs)
- Tegretol (Carbamepine)
- Phenobarbital
- Phenytoin (Dilantin)
- Primadone (Mysoline)

Because lithium is often the most effective treatment for manic depression or bipolar disorder, it's often crucial to stay on it even if it limits your penis's ups and downs.

THE IMPOTENCE PROBLEM

Antianxiety drugs in low doses among men who are anxious may actually help by reducing the anxiety that interferes with the parasympathetic nervous system's pointing mechanism. But they can also be impediments to sexual performance. Among the worst are:

- Oxazepam (Serax)
- Chlordiazepoxide (Librium)
- Chlorazepate (Tranxene)
- Diazepam (Valium, Valrelease)
- Meprobamate (Deprol, Equagesic, Equanil, Meprospan, Miltown), a terribly addictive alternative to other anxiety-blocking medications.

If you need a drug for anxiety, consider:

- Lorazepam (Ativan), which is from the Valium family, but spends only a short amount of time in your system
- Buspirone (Buspar), from a different chemical class than other anxiolytics

Antipsychotics may stop you from hearing voices, but you're not being paranoid if you suspect that they are sabotaging you in the sack:

- Prochloperazine (Compazine)
- Haloperidol (Haldol)
- Chlorpromazine (Thorazine)
- Chlorprothixene (Taractan)

- Thioridazine (Mellaril)
- Thiothixene (Navane)
- Fluphenazine (Permitil, Prolixin)
- Mesoridazine (Serentil)
- Promazine (Sparine)
- Trifluoperazine (Stelazine)

The new breed of antipsychotic medications fare far better where your phallus is concerned:

- Pimozide (Orap)
- Clozapine (Clozaril)
- Risperidone (Risperdal)
- Olanzapine (Zyprexa)

Street drugs act primarily through the central nervous system as psychiatric medications do. Although these drugs can all seem to increase desire and a sense of sensuality or intimacy, they ultimately all produce erectile dysfunction, not to mention ejaculatory impairment, in a high proportion of men who take them:

- PCP (angel dust)
- opiates (heroin, morphine, methadone)
- stimulants (cocaine, amphetamines, and methamphetamine or "crystal meth")
- psychedelics (LSD, MDMA or "ecstasy," MDA)
- volatile nitrites (amyl nitrite, or "poppers")
- marijuana
- benzodiazepines (Valium)
- barbiturates

Since Viagra's release, Pfizer has specifically alerted Viagra users to the serious drops in blood pressure that can occur when Viagra and amyl nitrite ("poppers") are taken together, because organic nitrites already cause smooth muscle vasodilation throughout the body.

Electrical Circuitry Problems

1. Brain
   - Lack of desire
   - Adrenergic outflow produced by strong negative emotions
   - Parkinson's disease and other neurological disorders
   - Psychiatric and neurological medications
   - Street drugs
2. Spinal Cord
   - Injuries due to accidents, tumors, strokes
   - Multiple sclerosis and other degenerative neurological conditions
3. Peripheral Nerves
   - Diabetes mellitus
   - Trauma
   - Surgery
   - Prostate resection
   - Bladder surgery
   - Colorectal surgery
   - Radiation treatment to pelvis, typically to prostate gland

The Physical Causes of Impotence

If you're like most mechanics, you like to know how things tick, to take them apart, examine what's wrong, and fix it. What I've shown you in the previous chapter and in this one is how your equipment works and what can go wrong with it. I've suggested that the power of Viagra lies in its ability to boost erectile functioning whatever the cause of the mechanical failure. But if your penis is the symbolic equivalent of a car, then your mind (and brain) is the driver. As you know, half of the car's performance depends on who's behind the wheel. Is the driver distracted, maybe fighting with a partner who's a backseat driver? Or perhaps the driver is rushing to get back to the office, screaming at his secretary on his cell phone. Before you respond to your erection problems by simply popping a pill, let's acquaint you with the mind of the driver who steers your penis during sex.

After all, it's the mind, not the penis, that's the most powerful sex organ in the body. Sometimes it's the mind that matters most.

3

The Psychological Causes
of Impotence

British race car driver Stirling Moss once said, "There are two things no man will admit he can't do well: drive and make love." He might have also said that driving and making love both involve style and panache, both use delicate, prized equipment, and both contain the potential for catastrophic crashes. In the previous chapters, we focused on the car itself— your sexual equipment and how it runs, as well as how it breaks down. We reviewed the three rods that make up your rod, discussed why one is spongy and how the cavernous ones work. We inspected the penile arteries, those fuel lines responsible for sexual turbocharging. We examined the neural wiring that allows you to point and shoot, get erect and ejaculate. We watched those sandbagging, well-coordinated chemicals up close as they worked frenetically to open the floodgates and create a blood flood that juices you up like gasoline hit by a spark. We saw that there's no shortage of reasons for mechanical failures with the equipment. And we learned a crucial fact: Because of its automatic, autonomic circuitry, once it's rolling, your penis has a mind of its own. You can hinder its efforts by getting anxious, or you can sit back, relax, and enjoy the ride.

Pioneering sexologists William Masters and Virginia Johnson were the first to study the sexual response cycle in men and women in a scientific way, setting up a lab to study the human sexual response in detail. Their lab had machines for electroencephalograms (EEGs, which trace brain waves), electrocardiograms (EKGs, which look at heart function) and the first plethysmographs, devices for measuring the onset, duration, and firmness of erections. The lab even contained a kind of motion picture studio that made movies of penises strutting their stuff and vaginas twitching at the moment of orgasm. All these instruments were used to capture the anatomical and physiological correlates of sexual arousal and climax in both normal subjects and those with various sexual disorders, including erectile dysfunction. Prior to these studies people thought that men and women had very different sexual responses, but Masters and Johnson were able to demonstrate that, in fact, the stages of sexual response and the physiology of arousal were similar. While men had penile engorgement resulting in erections, women had vaginal lubrication and clitoral engorgement as an important indicator of excitement. Most of the changes in blood pressure, heart rate, and vascular tone were similar between men and women. Men and women may be driving very different equipment, but there is a lot of similarity in how it functions. Perhaps unable to find anyone else who knew quite as much about sexual response as each other, Masters and Johnson later married.

WHY YOUR GRAY MATTER MATTERS

Masters and Johnson left out one crucial step in sexual response. Their version of the sexual response cycle started with arousal, completely leaving out the fact that desire is a necessary precursor. In effect, they did what we did in the first two chapters of this section, kicking the wheels of the car's tires without examining why anyone goes car shopping in the first place. In their attempt to be scientific, they left out the psychological side of sex entirely.

Some who preceded Masters and Johnson, such as Henry Havelock Ellis and Sigmund Freud, understood that sex was about more than mere mechanics. As every man with erectile dysfunction knows, mechanics are only half the picture. Sigmund Freud knew that when he focused on the role of sexual urges and sexual frustration in the development of psychological symptoms and illness. He originally thought that coitus interruptus, in which the man pulls out before orgasm, which was widely used as a means of birth control in Vienna, was responsible for neurosis. Freud briefly entertained some pretty fantastic ideas about the connections between the nose bones and the sexual response. But he was the first to recognize the crucial importance of feelings and fantasies in how people felt about sex, emphasizing the fact that when our emotions and ideas are unacceptable to us, we can develop neurotic symptoms, including erectile dysfunction.

The success of the Kinsey reports in the mid-1940s shows that people thought about sex quite a bit. Most wondered if they were normal in terms of what they thought about and did in bed. The questions Kinsey asked focused on his subjects' fantasies and behaviors. One thing Kinsey brought out of the closet was homosexuality, which was much more prevalent in his report than anyone had ever suspected. Kinsey also found high rates of masturbation and ascertained that it was fairly unusual for women to have orgasms during intercourse without direct clitoral stimulation.

Helen Singer Kaplan brought fantasy and sexual response together, following in the footsteps of Masters and Johnson but emphasizing an all-important first phase of the sexual response cycle that was psychologically driven: desire. She also recognized that what was running through our minds during every moment in the sexual response cycle influenced our physiological reactions in profoundly important ways. A thought that comes to mind that feels prohibited, unsolicited, or makes you uncomfortable can shut down sexual interest no matter where you are in the cycle. Kaplan pioneered the field of sex therapy. She later married the founder of Toys 'Я' Us. Apparently, they both knew how to have fun.

The sexual response cycle is the most pleasant almost-all-uphill trip you'll ever take. It all begins with desire—the drive to seek an adventure or go on a journey. Desire is the key to making your motor turn over. As Samuel Johnson noted, "Some desire is necessary to keep life in motion."

The three stages of the sexual response cycle—desire, arousal, and orgasm—are linked. Desire, the first stage, is a crucial determinant of whether arousal will follow. To be biblical about it, it's important to know whether the spirit is willing before we can determine whether the flesh is weak—or merely hasn't been put to the test yet. Desire is a kind of bridge between mind and body. Those racy thoughts and strong feelings that highly charged sexual and

---

Sexual Response =

Desire +

Arousal +

Orgasm

---

emotional situations evoke are caused by patterns of neural firing in the brain. Those brain waves in turn signal the equipment below the belt to get ready to go. But thoughts and feelings are the key to starting the engine.

The brain gets turned on by five main sets of stimuli: First, there are physical sensations related to touch, like having your neck kissed or your penis stroked. Then there are external perceptual inputs such as seeing that cute neighbor's legs in her new high heels, smelling your lover's perfume, or watching that movie from the cordoned-off area at the local video store. Other alternatives include internally generated fantasies, flights of fancy that include something you'd like to try or something you'd consider doing. Memories of actual experiences (or variations on a theme, hybrids of what really happened and what you wish had happened), can also be evocative and sexually charged. Strong inner emotions and feelings, such as intense love or attachment to your partner, can also make you want to behave sexually.

Brain turn-ons

Physical sensations

Visual stimulation

THE IMPOTENCE PROBLEM

Internal fantasy

Memories of actual experiences

Strong positive feelings

Thoughts dramatically influence feelings, so if a fantasy inadvertently stirs up guilt, it may inhibit your ability to get and stay aroused. Usually more than one factor conspires to create a sense of desire and the beginnings of arousal. Your brain will send messages down to the nerve endings in your corpus cavernosum that get your nitric oxide flowing, and your erection will spring into action. As my old anatomy book puts it: "pre-coital activity of variable duration and intensity is usually required to establish a receptive psychological attitude before sexual response and congress can occur." Pretty racy, huh?

Erectile dysfunction is generally thought of as a disturbance of the arousal phase of the sexual response cycle. And although desire has been broken off as a separate stage, the two are actually highly entwined: You notice the girl on the bus who reminds you of the supermodel you'd love to meet. Noticing her is the result of some modicum of desire already there, a kind of desire that leads you to see the erotic possibilities in situations in everyday life. The visual stimulation combines with a sense of interest to start the steps leading to arousal. So if desire is not present, arousal will not follow. It all begins with desire. We'll discuss problems of libido as separate from psychologically based problems with arousal and erection, but keep in mind that in real life the two phases meld into one seamless experience.

Consider the role of desire in skiing. There's the lack of desire that means you never make it up the mountain in the first place. That's the sense in which we define and talk about sexual desire: lack of interest, failure to notice the erotic cues. And then there's a different degree of lack of desire that means you ski down that slope even though your heart isn't in it. Or you ski it, but you chicken out halfway and snowplow instead. In the sexual equivalents of these cases, you'd be said to have a disorder of arousal, but I believe it's actually desire that lets you go all out. Desire is not limited to getting your warm body onto the chair lift. Sure, if you never start the car, you'll never get where you're going. But if you're not engaged in the journey, you'll get less out of the whole trip. The trip is about much more than those brief but lovely moments of airborne delight as you go over the cliff that is orgasm.

TALKING TESTOSTERONE

If arousal and orgasm consist of neat neural circuits, like electrical wires neatly tacked to a baseboard, then desire is like the electrical wiring diagram for the New York City subway system. Convoluted, messy, and complicated, with wires crisscrossing this way and that. The complicated network of neurons that make up your mind ultimately influence those lower, neat neural circuits that make up your point-and-shoot apparatus. Sexual desire is anything but easy and automatic. Desire is manifest in forms ranging from sexual fantasies and dreams ("I'd like to go on a trip") to masturbation ("I'd like to go alone") to the initiation of sexual behavior with a partner ("Would you like to come with me?"). Desire is the most fickle and complicated aspect of our sexual response.

We tend to think of desire as drive, an animalistic, biological aspect of sex that's the driving force behind our behavior. Drive is only one of the complex marriage of biological, psychological, and social factors that make up desire.

Components of Desire =

Biological Drive (Testosterone-related) +

Psychological Fantasies and Wishes +

Sociocultural Beliefs and Prohibitions

BIOLOGICAL DRIVE

Biologically based drive, fueled by testosterone (in women as well as men), is the most straightforward of these three components of desire. Testosterone acts as a kind of limbic lubricant, telling you to take an erotic interest in the world around you, encouraging you to scope out the scene and consider the possibilities. Testosterone is behind that tingly genital feeling, that radar for sexual opportunities, that impulsive reservation at a posh hotel for the weekend. And while only a small amount of testosterone is needed in order to get aroused and erect, its primary function is to spur desire.

Although small amounts of testosterone are made in the adrenal glands that sit atop the kidneys in both men and women, most of the testosterone in men is made in—you guessed it—the testes. A woman friend, born and raised in New York, fondly recalls getting partial credit on her seventh-grade science test for writing that testosterone was made in "the balls." Outside of New York, that answer would have gotten her suspended. Testosterone production in the testes occurs in the following way: First, the hypothalamus of the brain tells the brain's pituitary gland to produce two substances, FSH and LH, which respectively stimulate sperm production and testosterone production, both in the testes. Any disruption of the message between hypothalamus and pituitary or pituitary and testes can create problems, like a game of telephone between brain and balls that's gone awry. Psychiatric disorders such as depression, which affect the chemistry of these brain areas, as well as endocrine diseases of the

63

hypothalamus or pituitary, can lead to reduced testosterone.

Chronic heavy alcohol use is perhaps the most frequent biologically based reason for decreased sexual desire: Alcohol damages the liver and the damaged liver causes the overly rapid chemical conversion of testosterone into estrogen, the female hormone. Like a henpecked husband, the male alcoholic begins to grow femalelike breasts and exhibits testicular atrophy, with reduced testicular size as his testosterone gradually breaks down. This chemical conversion of testosterone to estrogen means that there is less testosterone around to promote desire. The testes, damaged by drink, also shrink in size, a common physical sign of alcoholism. As the porter in *Macbeth* noted, alcohol "provokes the desire, but it takes away the performance." In the long term, as heavy alcohol use reduces your testosterone levels, it takes away the desire as well.

Testosterone can seem too low even if your blood levels of it are adequate when the testosterone receptors are blocked by chemicals other than testosterone. These chemicals may sit on the testosterone receptors, but they do not act like testosterone while sitting there. Meanwhile, they block testosterone from stimulating its own receptors, like a person who sits in your seat in the theater and then refuses to get up when you complain that the seat should be yours. Histamine-blocking drugs often taken for indigestion are notorious for blocking testosterone's receptors. These drugs, available over the counter without a prescription, include:

- **Famotadine (Pepcid)**
- **Cimetidine (Tagamet)**
- **Ranitadine (Zantac)**

Because these drugs attach themselves to the testosterone receptors and just sit there, they tie up the line between testosterone and the testes. So if you're saying "Not tonight, dear, I have a stomachache" too often and popping a pill, you may in effect be chemically castrating yourself.

Over-the-counter antihistamines, the substances found in cold remedies and allergy preparations, are also histamine blockers that sit on testosterone receptors. The prime offender is:

- **Diphenhydramine (the active ingredient in Benadryl)**

That means that Loratadine (Claritin) and Fexofenadine (Allegra) are the clear and happy choices for chronic allergy sufferers.

Other medications that interfere with your testosterone reception include those used to treat fungal and other infections:

- **Metronidazole (Flagyl, Satric)**
- **Ketoconazole (Nizoral)**

The medications that like to sit on testosterone receptors are a strange group.

Finally, low testosterone can be caused by castration (orchiectomy, the removal of the testicles), which is often performed in prostate cancer patients to reduce the testosterone made there that can fuel the growth of the cancer cells. Alternatively, androgen ablation, a kind of "chemical castration," is sometimes achieved through the use of testosterone-blocking drugs, including:

- Estradiol (Estrace)
- Leuprolide (Lupron)
- Flutamide (Eulexin)
- Goserelin (Zoladex)

These treatments often leave patients with reduced libido as well as problems with erectile functioning. Combined with the surgery and radiation treatments used for prostate cancer, these men have multiple reasons for having both desire and arousal problems.

Current treatments for prostate cancer (ranging from surgery to placing small radioactive pellets in the prostate gland to halt the tumor's growth) results in excellent (more than 80%) ten-year survival rates in many patients, but the treatments that cure it come at a very high price for many. Even the mildly testosterone-inhibiting drug Finasteride (Proscar)—which is used to treat benign prostatic hypertrophy, a normal age-related increase in size of the prostate gland that leads to difficulty urinating in older men—can cause interference with libido and potency. In a lower dosage and known as Propecia, Finasteride was recently approved as an effective treatment for male pattern baldness.

Sometimes other disease processes, such as HIV, destroy the testicular cells that make testosterone, thereby interfering with sexual desire. It seems grossly unfair that those men unfortunate enough to be stricken with prostate cancer often get a chemical treatment that's also sometimes used with sex offenders such as pedophiles and rapists to decrease their sex drive. The only thing criminal about prostate cancer is the way it's rarely discussed and the fact that research on prostate cancer is underfunded.

My guess as a psychiatrist is that the only thing that makes men more anxious than the thought of having a life-threatening cancer is the idea that getting treatment for their condition can render their penises less capable. Cancer is enough of an assault on the self already without causing impotence, too.

If low testosterone levels are responsible for reducing your normally Latin libido, reducing drinking and limiting those medications likely to interfere (if possible) are important steps to restoring your sexual desire to its full potential. If testosterone levels are low due to normal aging, the midlife changes that Gail Sheehy has dubbed man-o-pause, then hormone replacement either via a transdermal patch (worn just like those used to stop smoking) or through semimonthly injections of testosterone may be indicated. In fact, a recent study demonstrated that testosterone levels drop 1% yearly between ages forty and seventy, for a 30% drop over those thirty years. Testosterone replacement can increase your libido, but it also raises your risk for prostate cancer. It can also inspire an increase in all those stereotypically male behaviors such as honking your horn too much or tooting your horn too often. Your partner may notice that if you were reluctant to stop and ask for directions before, you now absolutely and adamantly refuse. But even your frustrated wife, driving around in circles with you for hours, may conclude that it's a small price to pay to rekindle desire.

Our growing understanding of the gradual loss of testosterone of men in midlife will probably lead to hormone replacement for men. That replacement will have benefits in terms of sustaining men's interest in sex. But unless it's combined with a huge public campaign about the detection and treatment of prostate cancer (like the pink ribbon campaign for breast cancer) it will be a late-life health disaster.

PSYCHOLOGICAL FANTASIES AND WISHES

Unlike the biological component of sexual desire, which depends predominantly on testosterone, the psychological and social components of sexual desire are more complicated. They rely on myriad psychological factors within a person, between a person and his partner, and on sociocultural beliefs such as what constitutes appropriate sexual behavior. Though not driven by a fuel as simple as testosterone, these psychological and sociocultural forces and values nevertheless powerfully shape sexual desire.

Let's start with the psychology of the individual, with you. How do you feel when you let your mind run wild when you fantasize? Does it make you nervous? Many people are afraid to let their minds go, because they secretly know they won't like where they wander off to. What if you consider yourself a man's man but your mind keeps running off to boff inappropriate love objects? Fantasies can get us tied up in so many psychological knots that it sometimes seems simpler to lock them in the back bedchamber of our minds and throw away the key. But when we do, we imprison more than half our capacity for sexual excitement, fulfillment and enjoyment, like trying to drive a race car with your hands tied behind your back.

SOCIOCULTURAL BELIEFS AND PROHIBITIONS

Your inner psychological life as well as your partner's are in turn strongly shaped by religious ("Good Catholic girls don't"), ethnic ("All Italian men are studs") and cultural ("Red-blooded American men do it twice a day") beliefs about sex. Those beliefs can either help to whip up desire or take the wind out of your sails. Holding certain culturally based beliefs can also influence how thick the bars need to be to keep your free-wheeling mind in check.

Desire involves an integration of these biological, psychological, and social factors. But where do the psychological and social factors that shape desire come from? Desire is a reflection of your own core sense of sexual identity, the sexual vision of yourself that you forged during childhood and adolescence. So it's crucially important to getting sex revved up that your core sexual identity fit comfortably, like a well-tailored suit. Core sexual identity is composed of three main facets: gender identity, sexual orientation, and sexual intention.

Core Sexual Identity =

Gender identity +

Sexual orientation +

Sexual intention

YOUR SEXUAL CORE

The first aspect of core sexual identity is gender identity, that inner sense usually developed by two or three years of age that you are a girl or a boy and that that's exactly what you should be. Feeling that you're secretly trapped in the wrong body or failing to accept and ultimately relish your own sexual equipment will set you up for conflicts about what you desire.

Sexual orientation is the second major component of sexual identity and focuses on what gender of partner you prefer, same or opposite-sex. For many people, this choice comes as naturally as whether they prefer vanilla or chocolate, though for many gay people, deciding to admit to themselves or to others what they prefer may be difficult because of societal stigma. You may also find that you prefer to alternate between vanilla and chocolate and that you like them both, a sort of bisexual double-dipping. The content of your sexual orientation is less important here than your level of comfort with admitting whom you want sitting in the passenger seat beside you.

Finally, there's sexual intention, your sense of with whom (or what) you'd like to engage in sexual behaviors and what exactly you'd like to do. Sometimes sexual intention causes people difficulties because the object of their sexual desire is nonhuman, resulting in fetishes. How much of a problem this is depends upon both you and the object of your affections. If you find a patent leather shoe strapped in the passenger seat beside you, that's your business. If your fetish involves your pet poodle, that may be the ASPCA's business. But intentions toward human partners who are nonadult or nonconsenting can cause you messy moral and legal problems. You can seek out any unpredictable sexual passenger you like, assuming he or she is a consenting adult. Or you can decide it's simpler to travel alone in your auto erotic. Various sexual acts, too, can become obligatory or taboo. You can be as disturbed by your wish to engage in oral sex as you would be if you found yourself attracted to shoes.

Within the legal limits that apply to us all and the moral limits that each individual must define for himself, there is room for a wide range of sexual intentions. What really matters in terms of how your desires relate to arousal and erectile functioning is whether you accept and enjoy them, not what the images and wishes are.

This sense of your sexual self—gender, sexual orientation, intended partner, and choice of sexual acts—is core to shaping your desires and your inner fantasy life. But each of these areas can potentially become laden with psychological conflict, resulting in difficulties with your sexual functioning based on inhibitions, guilt about your desires, or the incorporation of angry or aggressive images into your sexual self. To make matters even more complex, your sexual self is not evolving in a vacuum, separate from the rest of you. Family dynamics shape your personality, which in turn determines how your sexual identity evolves.

PSYCHOLOGICAL BREAKDOWNS IN BED

Psychological problems arise from:

The presence of unacceptable fantasies
and feelings

Links between sex and past life
experiences, particularly aggressive ones

Mismatches between feelings and
fantasies and what you're actually doing

Mismatches between your and your
partner's core sexual identities

As we will see over and over again, when we address psychological issues involved in sexuality, there are four main ways that a driver can get into trouble, erotically speaking. First, having fantasies and feelings that seem unacceptable often leads to diminished desire and sexual inhibition, the inability to let yourself become aroused and reach orgasm. This psychologically based restraint of your penis is really an attempt to restrict your thoughts and feelings. You are anxiously trying to keep unacceptable sexual fantasies and emotions under wraps.

A second common psychological problem that contributes to problems of desire, arousal, and orgasm is that sex is linked in your mind to prior life experiences, often with parents, that involved aggression, anger, or other negative feelings such as guilt, disgust, or fear. Many of these revolve around issues of dominance and submission. In speaking of this type of dominance and submission, I am not referring to sexual sadomasochism à la the Marquis de Sade. What I really mean are power struggles between sexual partners, whether they occur in reality or in your mind.

A third problem of desire and arousal occurs when there are mismatches between what you're trying to do in bed and your core sense of self. Sometimes you may not even be aware of certain fantasies, though they may still stir up feelings and guide your behavior. And at other times, you may feel that you know you are masquerading in bed, pretending to be something that you wish you were. If you're secretly attracted to poodles and find that unacceptable, you will try to have sex with your partner instead. But the mismatch between desire and reality can contribute to sexual problems.

Fourth, when you add your partner's core sexual identity and desire into the mix, you can see why sex can become so complicated. Add a relationship with the ups and downs and pleasures and pressures of everyday life, and it's not surprising that sexual problems are so widespread. Freud believed that there are always more than two people in bed when we have sex because we carry early-life relationships and the fantasies they inspire around with us. It's an orgy, perhaps even a menagerie, psychologically speaking. All these factors affect your sexual desire and your capacity for arousal, whether you're male or female.

In the next chapter we'll look at how to tell the biological and psychological causes of impotence apart, taking into consideration that they're often intertwined. In addition, we'll discuss when determining the exact etiology of your erectile dysfunction matters, as well as what tests can help zero in on the cause.

4

Evaluating Impotence

The Viagra trials broke erectile dysfunction sufferers into two groups. The first are those with psychogenic or psychological reasons such as anxiety, lack of interest, or conflicts about power and dominance with their partners. Then there are those with organically based disorders such as atherosclerosis, nerve injury after prostate surgery, and diabetes. Those with psychological reasons for impotence tended to do better (84% general improvement in psychogenic group, compared with 43% of radical prostatectomy group and 57% in diabetes group). But Viagra was highly effective and easily used with few side effects regardless of the reason for impotence. There's a high proportion of patients whose impotence is mixed, the result of organic factors with psychological factors piled on top. This is not surprising, since impotence itself can induce anxiety about performance that is essentially self-defeating as well as a source of disturbances in important relationships.

Whatever the cause, Viagra is likely to help you overcome your erectile problems. Because it magnifies the usual sexual response cycle, it can take the tiniest amount of fuel and make your penis seem turbocharged in return. It can overcome damaged neural circuitry, within limits, whether the problem lies in the peripheral penile pathways or those intricate and complicated wires that make up the brain. Despite the well-worn warnings that it's not an aphrodisiac, Viagra can also boost a little desire into enough to get your penis fired up, given adequate physical stimulation.

But determining the cause of impotence still matters. Popping a Viagra may eliminate the problem, but your risk factors for atherosclerosis or your budding diabetes may be overlooked. If you don't understand the contributing causes, you may not be able to prevent your condition from becoming worse. Many of the medical dangers associated with impotence can be detected through good general medical care. Hopefully you get a general checkup at regular intervals anyway, complete with blood work. If you don't, and if you have erectile dysfunction, you should definitely get a checkup before you try Viagra.

Many men receive a cursory exam and a prescription with a slap on the back from their physicians and a "go to it" attitude. And that's just the kind of interaction about the drug that many men would prefer to have, since it doesn't delve too deeply into the sensitive problem of sexual dysfunction. It's probably the same psychology that led just 5% of men with erectile dysfunction to get help pre-Viagra. And while the new drug means the rewards of confessing that you've got a problem are larger, the fear, embarrassment, and concerns about tarnishing their "real man" images that men feel in discussing erectile dysfunction are certainly still at play. Sometimes, failing to take a comprehensive view of the problem can occur because your doctor is harried or pressed for time. After all, it's hard to write over 40,000 Viagra prescriptions a day, even with a rubber stamp. Another thing that may be overlooked in the rush to the prescription pad is that your problem may never be conceptualized as one of lack of desire, performance anxiety, problems in your sexual identity, or conflicts in your relationship with a partner. Overlooking these psychological conflicts, which are often amenable to individual therapy, couples therapy, or sex therapy, is a danger as well. Psychological symptoms have a wide range of complex and interconnected meanings, and simply overriding anxiety or anger with a pill can mean that the problems will fester. Remember: Viagra is a treatment for your penis. If it produces shifts in your problematic psychology as well, all the better, but sex depends on the car as well as the driver. Let's look at how to tell the two apart and what tests can be done to determine where your erectile dysfunction comes from. What follows is a kind of medical and psychological detective story that can give you a clue about the causes of your problem.

COLLECTING THE CLUES

Where was your mind the night the erectile dysfunction occurred? Was your penis with it? Putting the pieces of the puzzle together can require a top-notch detective. You should try to suss out whether it's the psychologically impaired Professor Plum or the organically impaired Colonel Mustard who's responsible for your problem before you consult your doctor. Trying to decide whether erectile dysfunction is psychological or physical may even guide your thinking about whom to call first—a urologist, internist, or psychiatrist.

The first step to determining the cause of your erectile dysfunction is to gather all the evidence.

Make as honest an inventory as you can of all the psychological motives you can find. Potential stressors that might interfere with your sexual functioning include:

- your current work situation and whether you are feeling angry or threatened about it
- financial, work-related, or family problems
- recent losses and setbacks
- factors that are making you feel less masculine
- your comfort level with your own body

- your comfort level with whom you're attracted to
- your comfort level with what you want to do in bed

Ask yourself some probing questions:

- Are your fantasies free and accessible or kept under lock and key?
- Are you so focused on performance that you find yourself anxiously anticipating failure?
- Do you feel angry, afraid, disgusted, repulsed by the thought of sex, either generally or with a given partner or sex act?
- Are you and your partner communicating well, or is there stress and tension, either about your impotence or about something else entirely?
- Do you feel your partner thinks that your erectile dysfunction makes you less of a real man?
- Have you been thinking about separating?
- Have you been having an affair, better sex with another partner where you are having adequate erections?
- Are there factors that are hindering intimacy, jeopardizing your ability to trust your partner?
- Are there factors that are making you feel unloving or unlovable?

Just because the answer to one or more of these questions is yes does not mean that these psychological factors are the main cause of your erectile dysfunction. Still, this psychological inventory provides an important context for understanding what's (not) up.

THE PSYCHOLOGICAL PROFESSOR PLUM

Certain clues would lead us to consider Professor Plum the prime suspect. If psychological factors are the primary cause of your impotence prior to the onset of erectile dysfunction, you would most likely be less interested in intercourse, have a shorter duration of coitus (often less than ten minutes) and report less-intense physical sensations (such as contraction of the muscles at the base of the penis). Sudden onset of erectile difficulties with a particular partner, sometimes combined with premature ejaculation, failure to maintain an erection until ejaculation, or difficulty reaching orgasm are other clues that would lead us to point a finger at psychological causes. When erectile dysfunction occurs consistently with specific sex acts but not with others (always with intercourse, for example, but never with oral sex), we can be highly suspicious of a psychological root cause.

Men with psychological causes for erectile dysfunction have normal erections during REM sleep, upon awakening, during masturbation, when stimulated visually by erotic materials, and often with new sexual partners. Men with psychological factors as the primary cause of their erectile dysfunction are also more likely to have partners who are critical of the problem and see it as evidence of lack of manhood. Interestingly enough, when men with psychologically based impotence were polled about the causes of their erectile dysfunction, they often said they believed that their impotence was either caused by or associated with psychological factors. If you want to determine whether Professor Plum is responsible, it might be as simple as just asking.

THE CAVERNOSAL COLONEL MUSTARD

The organically impaired Colonel Mustard, on the other hand, has a different historical presentation of his problem. The onset of his organic erectile dysfunction was generally more insidious and slow, as his hormone levels dropped from too much alcohol, or his arteries got narrower and narrower from too much fried chicken. Organic illness is often accompanied by reduced penile size due to the scarring of those delicate corpus cavernosum smooth muscle cells.

The exception to this rule about the gradual onset of impotence is impotence caused by a new medication or drug of abuse, a surgical procedure, or pelvic trauma, in which case the temporal relationship between the event and the dysfunction is usually clear and points to the cause. If the onset of erectile difficulties coincides with starting up on Prozac, that's the most likely source of your erectile problems.

Colonel Mustard's erections are likely to be less

regular and rigid at night and upon awakening than Professor Plum's. The good Colonel's erectile problems tend to affect him equally when he is masturbating, engaged in sexual acts other than intercourse, or having sex with a different partner. Sometimes when the excitement generated by sex with a new partner is very high, men with moderate erectile dysfunction will be able to have better erections than in other situations.

Men with organic causes of their dysfunction also have fewer sexual problems before the onset of impotence, with higher frequencies (greater than two times monthly) and longer durations (greater than ten minutes) of intercourse prior to the onset of the erectile problem as well as more pleasurable orgasmic experiences. They are less likely to have a history of premature ejaculation or decreased desire. Their sexual partners are unlikely to believe that their erectile disturbances make each of them less of a real man, and they are less likely to feel tension in their romantic and marital relationships, less likely to separate over the erectile dysfunction.

ASSESSING SEVERITY

Another aspect of erectile function that may require evaluation is its severity, which may be mild, moderate, or severe regardless of its psychogenic versus organic origins. Characterizing severity is important, because it helps to determine which treatments may work and how much they are likely to help.

Unfortunately, the less you actually need Viagra (or any drug) for impotence, the better it's likely to work for you. In severe erectile dysfunction, there may not be enough of the usual arousal response around for Viagra to magnify. Or, older treatments such as Caverject or MUSE (reviewed in the next chapter) may be more effective, since they deliver the medication directly to the penis. It's too early for comparison studies between the various agents to have been performed, so it's difficult to say how they'll stack up against each other.

An effective way to assess the problem, and one that your doctor may use, too, is the International Index of Erectile Functioning (IIEF). This self-report questionnaire will evaluate your erectile functioning, sexual desire, orgasmic function, intercourse satisfaction, and overall sexual gratification. Your doctor may use this test to evaluate your response to Viagra or whatever treatment for erectile dysfunction you ultimately opt for.

If you feel after reviewing these patterns that the cause of your impotence is likely to be psychological, you might first see a psychiatrist who can in turn help you decide whether other medical intervention is warranted. Some erectile dysfunction responds rapidly to psychotherapy or to specific sexual exercises, obviating the need for expensive medical tests and possibly even Viagra. But you may also opt for the benefit of an immediate response to Viagra combined with psychotherapy or sex therapy. The downside of this plan is that a psychiatrist generally does not conduct physical exams on outpatients and cannot address physical causes except by history, whereas an internist or urologist can talk to you (though with less understanding of what's happening upstairs), as well as examine you and conduct additional tests. But even if you feel more certain that the cause is likely to be organic in nature, you should try to be certain you'll feel comfortable discussing your problem with whichever physician you choose.

IN SEARCH OF THE CULPRIT

Of course, finding the cause of impotence is not so simple as deciding whether Professor Plum or Colonel Mustard is to blame. For starters, they might both be involved. Then there's the fact that there are many types of psychological and organic causes of impotence, the ones that we explored in Chapters 2 and 3. So whatever help you ultimately enlist, they'll probably use the schema I gave you in those earlier chapters for tracking down the cause. You will be examined for atherosclerotic risk factors: smoking, obesity, hypertension, high cholesterol, diabetes. The first three are readily attainable by your report and by a physical examination, including a blood pressure reading. Your cholesterol levels, which include overall cholesterol, triglycerides (fatty acids), HDL ('good" cholesterol), and LDL and VLDL ('bad" cholesterol) are easily checked from a blood sample while you're fasting. One recent study showed that high HDL levels are actually associated with good erectile functioning, perhaps even protective. So certain kinds of cholesterol can be your penis's friend.

Because diabetes can even present for the first time as impotence, your doctor will be asking questions about some of the subtle symptoms that can herald its onset: frequent urinating (which can also be a sign of a too-generous prostate gland), constant thirst, weakness, tiring easily, and weight loss are often early clues. Checking your blood glucose or sugar level while you're fasting and finding it at about 140 is practically diagnostic of diabetes. But if your ability to secrete and respond appropriately to insulin isn't clear from this simple test, you will be given a glucose tolerance test, in which you are given glucose and then examined for the rapidity with which you can lower your blood sugar. Your history of exercise may help your physician assess your overall level of health as well as what can be done to address your atherosclerotic risk factors.

In addition, other findings on your physical exam can assist your physician in determining how advanced your atherosclerotic disease or diabetes has become. For example, "cotton wool" spots on your retina can be signs of nerve damage from diabetes, or you may have the cool feet and lower legs typical of already partially blocked arteries or signs of coronary artery disease. Much as the penis is the ultimate focus of your attention, determining the cause of your erectile difficulty is a total body proposition. You wouldn't just examine the room where the body was found, would you? You'd check the whole house for evidence.

Other causes of arterial injury, such as trauma to the pelvic area in an accident or following pelvic or lower gastrointestinal tract surgery, are also possible reasons, often evident in taking a medical history but sometimes subtle. The same traumas and surgeries that cause arterial damage can also disrupt the delicate nerve networks in the area. So can any impingement on the spinal cord, even a back injury, or anything that disrupts the wiring along the way. Again, these potential problems are largely determined by history and physical exam. Neurological disorders of the brain and spinal cord such as Parkinson's disease or multiple sclerosis must also be suspected on the basis of history and physical exam. Some doctors are likely to be more thorough about looking for these factors than others.

Your history of drinking and drugs is important, since alcohol ultimately reduces testosterone and therefore sexual desire and performance, while most recreational drugs impair erectile capacity. Don't expect a Breathalyzer test, but be forewarned that this part of the picture requires honesty on your part to present an accurate portrait of your substance-use patterns. Your current medication regimen, especially those cardiovascular and psychiatric medications we discussed in Chapter 2, is equally important in determining the cause of your problem.

THE FORENSIC EVIDENCE

Now it's time for the real forensic examination, a look at the physical evidence. First, the basic blood chemistries—including a fasting blood sugar and a lipid profile (total cholesterol, triglycerides, HDL, LDL, VLDL) as well as a complete blood count—will check basic aspects of your physical functioning. It will also help to rule out risk factors for atherosclerosis. Although low testosterone is an unlikely cause of erectile dysfunction and more often results in reduced libido, testing testosterone levels as well as checking to see whether FSH, LH, and Prolactin levels (those messengers from the hypothalamus to the testes) are appropriate may also be warranted. If there are hints of any other (relatively rare) endocrine diseases, more specific endocrine tests may also be warranted.

Then there are tests to help your doctor determine whether the cause of your impotence is psychogenic or organic. Again, it's important to keep in mind that many men's problems are caused by some of both and that the psychological problems are ultimately brain-based anyway. Let's say it's nighttime and you've snuck into a room in which Professor Plum and Colonel Mustard are sleeping. If you've been paying careful attention to what I said earlier about how to tell the two apart, you know that one quick way would be to test for nocturnal penile tumescence: Who gets it up when his eyelids are down?

These tests revolve around harnessing the natural erections that occur during REM (or dreaming) sleep in males from under one day to over one hundred years old. The erections produced during REM are not the result of sexy dreams but rather a reflection of the fact that the parasympathetic nervous system prevails during dreaming sleep. Nighttime erections are unaffected by sexual abstinence or indulgence but they are interfered with by disruptions of the sleep-wake cycle, such as those due to psychiatric illnesses like depression. These tests have a certain intuitive appeal, because they give us a chance to examine the naturally occurring biological process of erections noninvasively, a chance to look at the operation of vascular, neural, and endocrine mechanisms with a minimum of psychological interference. After all, when you're asleep there's a greatly reduced chance that the hyperadrenergic tone produced by fear, anxiety, anger, or moral repugnance or disgust about sex will interfere with your erections. And even if it would, the powerful parasympathetic tone of the dreaming part of the sleep cycle would probably prevail.

Thus, failure of normal REM-related noctural penile tumescence indicates an organic component to your troubles, be it reduced testosterone, vascular problems, or nerve disorders. So if you snuck in and examined the Professor and the Colonel, you'd find

Professor Plum is the one who's sporting the largest banana, in his dreams, anyway.

There are three quick-and-dirty ways of testing for nocturnal erections and then a more high-tech (and high-cost) method. First is the so-called postage stamp test, in which you put a ring of postage stamps securely around your soft penis before bedtime. If the ring of stamps is broken in the morning, you have at least some nocturnal erectile functioning. Then there's the unfortunately named Snap-gauge, which you're supposed to wrap around your penis at night like the postage stamps and velcro shut. If the "teeth" (tiny plastic strips) of the Snap-gauge have snapped in the morning, your penis was rowdy the night before. Or else you thrashed about so much that you broke the stamps or snapped the teeth of the gauge. Even when these methods accurately reflect penile functioning, they tell you nothing about the number and duration of erections, or the degree of rigidity of the penis during the night— only that there was some tumescence (defined as a change in penile circumference).

Another possibility is to ask your willing partner to stay awake all night and monitor your manhood's whereabouts at all times. Obviously this requires dedication on her (or his) part, but it can give you a better sense of how many erections you have (most men have three to six) as well as how long they last and how firm they are. A psychiatric caveat: Since getting these nocturnal erections means that the cause of your potency problems while awake is generally psychologically based (or adrenergically, if you prefer), you'll need to consider how your partner will feel, sitting there all night potentially watching you get erections alone when you can't seem to do it together. (You'd better plan a nice dinner or flowers after this trying test.)

Then there's the RigiScan, the gold standard when it comes to nocturnal penile tumescence. It's expensive, requiring a one-to-three-night stay in a sleep lab. It's cumbersome, since you're being monitored with a band around the base and near the head of the penis as well as having eye movements and brain waves tracked. Once you have an erection, be prepared for a rude awakening: A technician will wake you up when your tumescence is maximal and apply an increasing amount of force to the head of your penis until it buckles, bending and bowing in response. Ouch. Rigidity refers to the pressure at which this buckling occurs. It is what determines whether your erection will be adequate for vaginal penetration. After that your penis will be photographed and inspected, rated and recorded. So you'll know whether your potency problem is psychological or organic. But even if the test is clearly negative (i.e., erections are absent), you still won't know what the cause of the organicity is.

A more economical way of assessing erectile functioning is to determine whether you can actually get an erection in response to a penile injection of a vasodilating substance. If you do, your erection can then be evaluated for duration and quality. (As you can guess, these "tests" in which men's members are evaluated and judged, which they can pass or fail, wreak further havoc with their already pounded self-esteem.) The rationale for the use of intracavernosal injections can be threefold. First, they help your doctor determine whether the vascular, neuronal, and endocrine mechanisms required for erection are intact. Second, they may indicate whether such injections are a permanent potential treatment for your problem. Third, it is vastly reassuring to many men, despite the potential pain of the injection itself, to see that they can indeed have an erection.

Sometimes your physician will opt to give you such an injection and then study blood flow to the penis with either penile plethymyography, a duplex Doppler, which is an ultrasonic, radarlike device that determines how fast your blood flow is going, whether it is speeding or not. In this case the erectile police are looking for Sunday drivers, blood that's just meandering along your penile superhighway rather than gunning down those arteries like a bat out of hell. Atherosclerosis and diabetes are the most common reasons for Sunday driving.

Other tests are more commonly used if your physician is considering surgery to cure your impotence. For instance, penile arteriography—which involves the injection of dye into the arteries to visualize blockages on X ray—will let your doctors know where the problem is. If there is a high suspicion that a veno-occlusive problem is the cause of your difficulties, your physician may even infuse saline into the corpus cavernosum. This produces a "water-based" erection that's as rigid and full as possible. Then your doctor can watch its efflux to see whether your veins shut down properly when fully compressed within the corpus cavernosum.

Another alternative is to inject dye and then X-ray the region to determine whether the dye flows out of the penis via the veins at an inappropriately fast rate. But rest easy, because normally there's no need for such shenanigans unless you're contemplating vascular surgery for a venous problem. Continuing this tour of medical tortures, it's also technically possible to put needlelike electrodes into your penile nerves and study nerve conduction or to test the autonomic nervous system more generally for dysfunction with the acetylcholine sweat-spot test. Luckily, most physicians and their patients lack a sweet spot in their heart for these heartless tests, which do little to improve the clinical management of nerve dysfunction anyway and are reserved for research purposes.

Viagra may reduce the need for some aspects of detective work. If it works, it's a real question as to how far to pursue the issue of exact diagnosis. At a minimum, a thorough evaluation including blood work and a head-to-toe physical examination may suffice. But Viagra won't work for everyone, so you may still have a need to determine the cause of your erectile problems to help you and your doctor decide what constitutes the best alternative treatment.

PART II

The Viagra Solution

5

Contemplating Viagra: Case Studies

By now you can understand the physical and psychological problems that arise when the penis fails to rise to the occasion, if you haven't already experienced them firsthand. When couples cope with impotence, there are some common patterns to how they try to deal with it: Denial tops the list, with everyone tiptoeing around the large pink elephant in the bedroom and pretending not to see it. We usually use denial when a subject arouses anxiety or is perceived as a threat. This chapter will examine the reactions of men with impotence and their partners, as well as what kinds of communication about their impotence issues evolved. Through their stories we'll see in detail some of the main psychological themes that recur.

Rob and Jill

My patient Rob is a handsome sixty-four-year-old man married for over forty years to his wife, Jill. He ran a large company that he started in his early twenties and built into a successful manufacturing firm. He was forced to retire because of atherosclerotic heart disease that produced frequent chest pain. The heart disease was also the cause of his impotence. His erectile dysfunction began to occur when he was in his late fifties and became increasingly severe over time.

Rob came to psychotherapy complaining of depression. His opening line in therapy was predictable: "I hate to say it, because intellectually I know better and I think it sounds juvenile, but I really do feel like my potency problems mean that I'm just not man enough." He responded well to Prozac, and it did not seem to produce any change in his level of erectile dysfunction. As his mood improved, he began to work in psychotherapy on his feelings about the interplay of power and dominance with penile functioning and impotence as well as to explore his reactions to aging.

Rob's first attempt to handle how he felt about his impotence was to have an affair with a younger woman. Although his wife never learned of it, Rob felt intensely guilty because he really loved his wife, whom he'd married at the end of college. He performed better with his new partner, but ultimately terminated the relationship, feeling that an affair was not the answer to his potency problem. Over time his sex life with Jill became more and more infrequent and constricted. But their channels of communication remained open and they enjoyed cuddling and kissing in bed. It was obvious in my work with them that they loved each other, and they showed little evidence of the power struggles that dominate many couples' daily lives.

One day Rob reported the following dream: "I'm at my golf club and I'm taking a lesson from the club pro. I keep swinging at the balls and missing them, one by one. And when I do hit them, they dribble just a little bit away from me and I can't seem to find them again. The pro keeps telling me how to do better, but I can't. I see Jill sitting outside with a man I used to play golf with and I get intensely angry and envious. I know I could have whipped him on the course before, but now I'm not so sure."

Rob quickly recognized his problems with his golf swing as a representation of his potency problems. He related the dribbling and loss of golf balls in the dream to his less powerful stream of urine and his sense that his testes were smaller than they used to be. He was surprised to find how angry he was at Jill for being with the other man in his dreams, even after he woke up. He knew it wasn't her fault, of course. After all, it was *his* dream. But it had real emotional resonance for him anyway. He said, "I look around at the club and think about how many men could beat me at golf now. I always looked forward to retiring and playing every day, but I'm just too physically ill to do well now. I still have days when I feel like, damn it, I should be able to drive my penis just the way I used to be able to drive the ball down the green. And I used to be able to drive myself in other areas as well. I was good at working faster, better, harder, longer. My penis should be able to keep the pace, too." Sometimes Rob imagined that after he died, Jill would still be hanging out at the clubhouse, dating other men, perhaps relieved to find someone whose golf swing was still strong. The thought was torturous, intolerable. But worse was the thought of leaving Jill alone, knowing that she was quite dependent on him.

"I also feel angry that it's in part my view of myself as a man that produced my problems in the first place. If I hadn't bought into that 'real man' stuff, I might not have worked such long hours, eaten red meat like it was going out of style, and drunk like a fish. I did make it to the top, but there was always someone just a little bigger anyway, some guy with a little more power or money. Don't get me wrong, though. It's not like I didn't enjoy it. I got off on the power and success, the awards and watching my net worth climb. But the problem with the equation of masculinity and power is that it's inevitable that your power will wane one day. But now, the fact that I'm not working, can't be active because of my heart disease, and can't make love to my wife because I can't get it up makes me feel like I've been demoted."

As treatment continued, Rob began to talk to Jill in a new way. And he confessed to me: "It's not that having impotence has been all bad, you know. It's meant I have to learn to talk to my wife, to try new things in bed, to confront my own feelings about getting older and more fragile physically and phallically. I've even come to enjoy Jill more in bed, getting to know her body and what pleases her that doesn't involve intercourse. And it led me to get into treatment with you. I've recovered some access to my inner feelings about things, to how many years I've spent feeling secretly inadequate while appearing to be such a clear-cut success on the surface. And I suppose that because we've been talking about sexual fantasies, you've given me more permission to think about them during sex. So I guess that makes you the pro in the dream," Rob laughed.

For Rob, impotence was equated with aging and death. "I'm sixty-four. With all my medical problems, I have to conclude that I'm probably near the end of my life. Every machine breaks down sooner or later. I intend to spend my remaining years trying to be more man than machine. But it's often still hard not to see myself as broken, less of a man. I miss being able to make a hole in one."

Jill concurred with Rob's assessment of the impact of impotence on their lives together. "Sometimes," Jill said, "I really miss the feeling that Rob is invincible, always able. It's made me understand how much I depend on him and it's made me feel a bit guilty for all the pressure I've inadvertently put on him over the years. I really miss having him inside of me, too. But I do think there's been a clearly positive side to the problem, meaning that it's forced him to challenge his definitions of what manhood means. I like having a partner who's more of an equal, and in fact we enjoy each other more now than ever." It was interesting to me (though certainly not uncommon) to see that as we worked together on these issues for a few sessions, Rob's potency problem—although it was clearly based in large part on medical factors—began to improve.

The couple had considered penile implants and Rob had briefly tried injections to produce erections, but they had concluded that neither the elaborate surgery (risky, given Rob's cardiovascular health) nor the injections that made Rob squeamish were worthwhile. But when I told Rob and Jill about the impending release of Viagra, they were nevertheless eager to be first in line. "It's not that I want to be eighteen again," Rob stated. "I mean, I like having the mind of a sixty-four-year-old, the insights I've gained through this problem. But that doesn't mean I wouldn't enjoy a new sports car if one's available. I'd be a far better driver than I ever could have been at eighteen. After all, my identity isn't centered in my groin anymore. My penis doesn't define me as a real man. But it'd still be fun to have a new and improved model. I'd like to take it out for a spin." For her part, Jill laughed and said, "I'm ready to give it a whirl, too, as long as I'm certain that it's still the Rob I've gotten to know better and come to love more during this difficult period who's at the wheel. But I have to confess that I worry about whether he will retain what he's learned when his new Maserati actually arrives. I'd almost like to have the prescription written out to me so that I could control how he uses it. Like making your teenage son ask for the car keys when he wants them." Speaking of sons, Rob's coming to terms with his potency problem had an unexpected benefit: After much wrangling about letting his son take over his company completely, Rob finally gave up control. And he said he was determined to convey to his son what he'd finally learned when he developed erectile dysfunction about what was really important in life.

JIM

There were many times I wished that Jim, a twenty-eight-year-old with a fast-track Wall Street career who had recently completed his MBA, were Rob's son. He, too, needed to learn the lesson that Rob had finally learned late in life about what being a man means. Jim was not in a relationship and he did not technically have erectile dysfunction. He seemed to me to be working overtime to fend off feelings that he was not a true man. He had massive amounts of anxiety about whether he was good enough that had interfered with his sexual performance on two occasions with two different women. It seemed that no summer home, no car, no bank account could quite be enough to satisfy Jim, to make him feel secure. It seemed clear to me that he had bought into the same image as Rob had many years earlier of what makes a man. I almost wanted to introduce the two (although as a psychiatrist I would never actually do such a thing), to give Jim a clear message about where he was headed if he didn't work on the underlying issues involved.

There was no evidence that Jim was gay, as he had no sexual fantasies about men, but he often worried that others at work would think he was. He had bought into the societal equation that weakness means you're not a dominant, assertive real man, which therefore means you're a weak, passive woman, which means you're a homosexual.

Jim's real problem was that he was self-centered: He had never outgrown the notion that he and his penis were the center of the world. Although he had little trouble getting dates, women often refused to see him a second time. He'd heard about Viagra from a market watch of Pfizer stock. He was certain it was what he needed to gain absolute control over his penis, his masculine identity, and thus his anxiety.

As his physician, I had no intention of prescribing it to him, believing that he had no medical need for it and that it would only reinforce his theory that sexual performance was paramount. I felt sure he'd easily get it anyway, but I wanted to see the normative steps in male adolescent development unfold in his psychotherapy. I believed that Jim was stuck at a kind of adolescent stage, which many men go through in the late teens and early twenties, in which they are focused on beating and competing, on whose penis is longer and on who's getting the most sex. For most men continued psychological development in their twenties and thirties results in a gradual delinking of self-esteem and phallic power, a kind of spreading out of the identity over the entire body rather than centering it in the groin. This shift in identity is often the result of meeting one's life partner and establishing a loving sexually fulfilling relationship. It is one of the best-kept secrets of many men's lives that they are tremendously fulfilled by their emotional connections to their wives. She is often the first real confidant with whom they can make increasingly long forays into vulnerability without expecting disaster or humiliation. This relationship may be the closest many men ever come again to returning to the days when their mothers were central in their lives and when being vulnerable was acceptable, even expected. No amount of Viagra could help Jim have a fulfilling sex life if it continued to revolve solely around his penis.

BILL AND JANINE

Bill and Janine each had their own sexual problems, and their relationship was troubled as well. I treated Janine in individual psychotherapy for several months before suggesting we meet with Bill. She came to treatment to talk about whether to leave him, but was hesitant because of their two children, both in their teens. Sex with Bill had never been ecstatic for Janine. She had never had an orgasm during intercourse, although she could reach one when masturbating, and she felt that Bill was really not interested in her sexual pleasure. He was unwilling to consider cunnilingus, for example. She was concerned that her lack of responsiveness meant she was frigid. Bill had a tendency to reinforce this fear in her by implying that past partners had no problem with how he made love.

Bill's problems with erectile dysfunction had begun three years earlier, when he began drinking more heavily. Bill's reaction was to withdraw from initiating sex. Janine took Bill's impotence as a sign that Bill didn't really love her any longer and wasn't very attracted to her, and she blamed herself for gaining weight. His erectile dysfunction made her feel like less of a woman, as if his penis was a literal peter-meter of her attractiveness and desirability as a woman. She was hurt and angry, though she tried to cover it up by acting overly sympathetic to his plight. Bill felt belittled by her sympathy, babied in a way that often made him go ballistic. It was frequently her expressions of sympathetic understanding ("It's all right, I don't think less of you as a man" or "It's not so important to me, we'll just cuddle instead") that touched off one of their many screaming matches. These fights ended with each saying horrible things to the other that they later regretted but secretly believed. Bill would point to Janine's weight gain as a reason for his lack of arousal, while she would suggest that the weight gain was a result of his erectile difficulties.

There were many more issues of power, dominance, and humiliation within Bill and Janine's relationship than within Rob and Jill's. These issues dated back to their early marriage, when Janine chided Bill about his less-than-stellar work performance in a way that was similar to the manner in which her own mother had humiliated her father. It seemed clear that Bill had gotten the message that he was a failure, a pathetic loser at work. Bill's thinly veiled hostility toward Janine's role as housewife and mother and his sense of entitlement to have whatever he wanted sexually speaking also came through loud and clear to her. "Suck my dick" was both a sexual demand and a means of expressing anger with Janine. Bill's anger was also manifest in the crude jokes about women he would frequently start our sessions with, apparently trying to establish dominance over me, dismissing me as just another "cunt" with whom he had to contend. The pair insisted in thinking of their problems as purely the result of sexual dysfunction, teaming up in their derision of me when I suggested they needed couples counseling.

Janine learned about Viagra while watching television and promptly told Bill. After he got over his initial huffiness at her suggestion that he try it, they both began to await the arrival of Viagra as if it were going to be a transformative religious experience, fixing years of marital discord and threats to separate. And I was alarmed by the degree to which Bill seemed to view it as his equivalent of the Bomb, the weapon that would "put the bang back in my banana," as he put it. I wondered if Janine heard the gun imagery that I did, with its undertones of violence. Although she did not express it directly, she seemed to sense it, saying that she was concerned about what Bill would be like with Viagra. It might make him more obnoxious than ever. Meanwhile, I worried about how Viagra might tip the always precarious balance of power in Bill's favor. As James Peterson, the "Playboy Advisor" columnist, recently said, "You can take an angry couple and give them Viagra, and then you'll have an angry couple with an erection."

BOB AND PETE

Then there were Bob and Pete, a gay couple for many years who were in their late sixties. Pete's prostate cancer and subsequent surgery a year before they came to see me put a damper on their usually active sexual life as well as producing emotional problems for them. With many of their peers dead from AIDS, the two really relied on each other, feeling that it was their love and the success of their relationship that had kept them both alive and able to cope with the loss of so many close friends. Though they occasionally engaged in sex with a third person, they were otherwise monogamous and clearly deeply in love.

One of Bob's reactions, in his terror that Pete might die, was to pull away and have an on-line romance with a partner he never actually met. Pete felt understandably hurt and the pair's enjoyment of nonsexual physical intimacy slowly cooled. He joined an Internet support group for men with prostate cancer and their partners, and it was there that he heard that Viagra was on the horizon. The support of his on-line friends was clearly helpful, but it still took time in therapy for both to understand that Bob's reaction of having an "affair" was less about Pete's impotence per se than his fears of losing Pete, his life partner.

There were also covert issues of competition between the two, about which both felt immensely guilty. Pete envied Bob's capacity for arousal even as he himself enjoyed and was the recipient of Bob's erect penis. And Bob was intensely guilty for enjoying being "the real man" in their relationship once again. Pete felt embarrassed when he used a vacuum pump to produce erections after surgery, often retreating to the bathroom and returning with an erection instead of using it in front of Bob. Bob tried to make the situation better by buying various cock rings for Pete, which in fact humiliated him further, even though he realized that the gifts were loving tokens and not intended to upset him.

Pete's impotence reawakened an old conflict in their relationship about who was on top sexually. As in many gay couples, the issue of who was the real man was fraught with difficulty. Uncovering Bob's fears of abandonment and revisiting the relationship issues they had resolved successfully years before got them cuddling more in bed and speaking more frankly about sex, love, and death. These talks prepared the way for Viagra to work by ironing out some of the problems between them in advance. The pair viewed Viagra as a tool that would help them reconnect, and enjoy their lives together.

CHRIS

Chris was a twenty-four-year-old student who came to see me for psychotherapy, stating that he had sexual troubles. He was sexually involved with a girlfriend he had been dating for about eight months who was beginning to talk seriously about their future in a way that made him nervous. He was about to graduate from college and trying to decide about his career, with mounting pressure from his parents to get "off the dole." Chris rarely initiated sex with Wendy, but when she attempted to interest him, he found himself focused on things that were wrong with her, finding her breath not fresh enough or her vagina "too smelly." He often had trouble achieving an erection. He even instructed her to douche daily and put on deodorant before bedtime. Chris was completely unaware of his inner fantasy life, though he did finally tell me his shameful secret: He liked to touch women's genitals on crowded buses and in the subway, and it was then that he could ejaculate without even touching himself. He had some interest in exposing himself to women as well but had been too afraid of getting caught to actually try it.

Chris was raised by his grandmother alone while his mother, who was a drug addict, was in jail. His grandmother demanded slavish affection from her young subject, and Chris was rewarded for being exceptionally good by being allowed to give her a scalp massage before bedtime. He remembered pushing his penis against the end of the couch until it hurt as part of the process, trying to guarantee that he would not get an erection. Chris read about Viagra's FDA approval in the newspaper and inquired whether I thought it could help him. He knew it wasn't supposed to be an aphrodisiac, but he hoped it might make him more interested in sex if he knew he could perform well. He was discouraged enough by his disgust with his girlfriend that he thought of breaking up. It was clear to us both that his sexual problems had a psychological basis, though, since he had no difficulty with erections while masturbating to erotic tapes. But even though he'd concluded from what he'd read that Viagra probably wouldn't help, he wanted to try Viagra anyway. He seemed to be depending on psychotherapy, not a drug, to really get to the root of his problems as a sexual man.

TOM

When Tom came to treatment, he was demoralized and distressed. His fiancé had recently broken their engagement after he was involved in a serious cycling accident that left him with some memory impairments as well as an injury to his pelvic nerves that impaired his potency. Tom had always been active and vigorous, but now multiple fractures in the accident had put a damper on his athletic interests and abilities. He felt sidelined. It was uncertain, since the injury had happened only four months earlier, how much of Tom's erectile dysfunction would clear up as some of his nerves repaired and regenerated themselves. Tom's main problem was difficulty sustaining an erection during intercourse, when he kept getting "soft" again despite intense feelings of excitement. Tom heard about Viagra from his physical therapist, Cindy. Though she did not specifically know that erectile problems were an issue with him and did not ask, she did mention that many of her patients with spinal-cord injuries were eagerly awaiting its approval. Tom didn't know much about the medication, but when he asked me about it I reassured him that there was indeed a good chance that it could help his erectile dysfunction.

But even if he recovered from his injuries, nothing could bring his fiancé back. Tom felt "burned," as he put it, by her sudden desertion, as if his basically trusting instinct had been undermined in a crucial manner. Part of the work of the therapy was to repair this ability to trust another woman, as well as exploring what turned out to be the considerable negative sides of his relationship with Ellen. It turned out that she had a dramatic flair for provoking fights from which evolved tearful reconciliations and confessions of undying love. The sex following these fights was better than ever and sometimes involved Tom's playfully restraining her. Tom knew that Viagra couldn't make him trust again, but he was excited about the idea that Viagra might help his erectile problem until it became more clear how much of his nerve function would return to normal as his injury faded to a distant memory.

JANE

Jane was a thirty-five-year-old woman who had been in psychotherapy with me for several years. Her relationship with her boyfriend, Arthur, was in crisis after three years. Among the issues were her partner's overly dependent manner and his expectation that Jane be the more active and assertive one in bed. Jane had a lifelong history of depression and had been on Paxil for several years to good effect, including an increase in her interest in sex. But since the troubles with Arthur had begun, she required a higher dose, just enough to make it impossible for her to reach orgasm except when using a vibrator on a high setting. She'd also noted less vaginal lubrication despite high levels of excitement, which decreased her pleasure and comfort during vaginal penetration. And trials of other antidepressants simply hadn't worked as well as her Paxil had. Jane was feeling resigned but deeply frustrated when I told her that many of my colleagues seemed to think that Viagra might help women as well. Although she had reservations about taking one pill to counter the effects of another, she was excited about the possibility and promptly began to research who would be conducting the clinical trials of Viagra in women.

Each of these patients and their partners began the Viagra countdown, ready to be first out of the gate to try the new wonder drug. For Rob, the drug represented a shiny new sports car driven by a more mature driver. For Jim, it represented a kind of ego glue for a fragile, traditional male identity that he wanted desperately to consolidate. For Bill, a lethal weapon to turn the tide in his favor in his lengthy marital battle. For Pete, a way to reconnect within his relationship. For Chris, the slim hope of short-circuiting years of intensive psychotherapy. For Tom, a chance to get on with his life after a serious injury. And for Jane, a way to circumvent the sexual problems Paxil had produced. I waited for one of the most widespread experiments in pharmacological history to unfold in my office. Given all the complexities of masculine identity, the psychology of the penis, and the meaning of impotence, I was in a unique position to see what the pill could provoke in my patients' minds and relationships.

The erection, seemingly the main event, was actually the least of it, in my mind. After all, a drug that worked in almost 80% of patients was bound to create forty million identical sound bites: men saying simply, "It worked!"—perhaps with something about feeling eighteen again thrown in for good measure.

But as a psychiatrist, it was the pillow talk that followed the pill that really interested me. There's an old saying, a quote by Bishop Mervyn Stockwood, that says that a psychiatrist is someone who "goes to the Folies Bergère and looks at the audience." As a psychiatrist, I would now have a chance to find out how much a pill that practically guaranteed erections could actually make people want to have sex again. As many people wanted to see Viagra's rise as Niagara Falls, but to me what might happen downstream promises to be equally powerful.

6

Viagra in Action: Case Studies

Viagra may be the one exception to the general rule that we are bored by pictures of other people's safari vacations. In part, the Viagra phenomenon has been fueled by word of its high rates of efficacy, but it's also created an unprecedented kiss-and-tell phenomenon, in which people test-drive the drug and then talk about it. This chapter will detail how Viagra works, highlighting why it has the effects and side effects it has. But Viagra's chemistry, while important to understand, is not where the real interest lies. So this chapter will also show you what Viagra has done for my patients.

Some of the stories you'll hear are from men who wrote to me in response to inquiries about their— and their partner's—experiences on the Internet. If you're a Viagra virgin, chances are you'll feel that same rush of excitement you felt when you looked at the pictures of male and female anatomy in your science books or sneaked a peek at that dog-eared copy of that smutty novel.

A Real Drug

Viagra started out in life as the lowly UK-92480, a.k.a. Sildenafil citrate. Even back in 1996, when its journey began, it was already a highly competitive and super-selective inhibitor of phosophodiesterase, which could inhibit the action of the villainous PDE5, which you'll remember breaks down the ever-popular cGMP, the penile powerhouse that loosens up smooth muscle cells and creates an erection. It became clear that if Viagra could beat PDE5, it would be a hero worldwide.

But Viagra was misunderstood. The folks at Pfizer just didn't understand its specialty, PDE5. They wanted it to inhibit PDE3, the subtype of phosphodiesterase found in the coronary arteries. They were, in effect, asking a high jumper to run hurdles instead.

The Pre-Viagra Era

Fred Flintstone (not his real name), forty-five, had been battling impotency for four years when he first took Viagra as part of a Pfizer clinical trial for the atherosclerosis that was to blame for his chest pain as well as his problems below the belt. As he downed his first dose, Viagra raced through his arteries and veins, looking for its nemesis, PDE5, and locating it down below Fred's belt. Within sixty minutes, Viagra's level had peaked in Fred's blood, its strength reduced by that high-fat brontosaurus-burger Fred had eaten as well. Viagra was about 96% bound to its host, forced to travel around his bloodstream, attached to proteins that functioned as tour guides. Less than .001% of it was able to sneak off into the semen undetected.

As it reached the liver, Viagra was broken down by the Cytochrome P450 army, especially component 3A4 and its assistant, 2C9. The Cytochrome P450 system is responsible for the metabolism of all sorts of drugs, a highly specialized army that cleaves medications chemically, breaking them into component parts. At times, breaking drugs down inactivates them and at other times it produces active metabolites, offspring of the parent drug that carry on its mission. When Viagra was split apart, its slightly altered (N-desmethylated) offspring was almost a chip off the old block. Viagra's N-desmethylated version was about 50% as potent as Viagra in terms of its ability to block PDE5. It had concentrations in the bloodstream of approximately 40% of those seen for Sildenafil itself. So Viagra's offspring would ultimately account for 20% of Viagra's effectiveness in defeating PDE5.

Within four hours, half of Viagra was gone, 80% through Fred's feces and the rest pissed away in Fred's urine. But before its demise, Viagra had made itself known to Fred and his wife. Less than an hour after Fred swallowed the pill, his once-mopey dick began to stir. Even though Fred had chest pain while having sex with Wilma, he persevered. It was the first time since they'd moved to Bedrock that the Flintstones felt the earth move. Fred felt he had to tell Pfizer what Viagra had done for him and his marriage.

THE MODERN ERA

Rob, the sixty-four-year-old who wanted his golf swing back was one of the first to get the drug when it was released. His urologist had written him a prescription about a week before the drug was actually FDA-approved. On March 27, he and Jill began to call all over town in search of a pharmacy that had it in stock. All around New York signs saying "We have Viagra" or simply "Viagra" began appearing in pharmacy windows as the stampede began.

I saw Rob the afternoon before he was to test-drive Viagra for the first time. He was excited but anxious. He'd placed so much hope on the pill. What if he was in the 20% that Viagra didn't help? That fascinating session essentially amounted to a back-and-forth struggle between the side of Rob that desperately wanted the medication to work and the side that kept reminding himself of all that his potency problems had taught him, the eighteen-year-old and the sixty-four-year-old struggling for control. "If it works, I'm buying a new sports car," Rob informed me. "Viagra sounds like the name of a sports car anyway, something you'd sell to aging baby boomers like me. I can see the ad now, a purring female voice saying, "Test-drive the all-new Viagra. It'll take you from sixty-four to eighteen in no time flat.""

"On a more serious note," I said, countering Rob's levity, "tonight's a big night for you. So good luck with it." I was a bit at a loss as a psychiatrist to know what to say about test-driving Viagra. "Good luck" was my stock phrase for patients facing all kinds of life challenges between sessions, my way of indicating that I wished my patients well, that I was on their side. I figured it would have to do for Viagra, too. Hearing myself say it to Rob was the first time I noticed my own feeling about the drug: If it did what it looked like it would do, it would change the lives of so many men like Rob. All the jokes about the need for "commitment pills" and about men acting like irresponsible teenagers aside, I knew that most men were not the two-dimensional lug-heads they were often portrayed as being. Though there was a comic element to the "real" men jokes, I really believed that it was society, all of us, who had conspired to make men judge themselves by the success of their penile performance.

When I saw Rob the following week, he'd brought Jill along. They were both smiling as they entered the office. "Well?" I said. "It worked!" they replied together. "I had a bit of that blue haze over my vision, that film that everyone talks about. And I turned beet-red in the face. But it was worth it." I suggested to Rob that he consider trying 50 mgs instead of the maximum dose of 100 mgs next time, thinking that it might work just as well, with fewer side effects.

For Jill's part, she reported that she'd never had better sex, because Rob had a stronger erection and kept it longer. We had talked previously together about the fact that women's and men's sexual responses were on different timetables, even when men's potency was not an issue. But with Rob getting a full erection not long before ejaculation, there had previously been practically no chance that Jill would reach orgasm during intercourse. In fact, she never had earlier in their marriage, either. "I never realized it before now," Jill said. "It's not the length in inches but the length in minutes that counts in terms of pleasing women." Rob smiled as Jill continued, "I did have concern at one point, looking at Rob huffing and puffing on top of me, about whether he'd have a coronary on the spot." I told Jill that indeed intercourse is physically quite strenuous and that the same rules apply to sex as other cardiovascular workouts. As it says on the top of the StairMaster, "stop if you feel lightheaded, short of breath or experience pain."

"Well, for my part," Rob rejoined, "I think feeling more manly will make me more inclined to try to get back in shape. I feel almost embarrassed admitting to you both that that's how I feel, as if after all this talking and work with you both, I should be over it." With this statement, Rob became my first patient with "Viagra guilt," a kind of apologetic deprecation of his own enjoyment of erections that I would see in other men as well. I imagined that the "It's not the Viagra that really got me going, it's you" line could not be far behind. I wondered how women would respond as they realized that a pill could do what they could not.

On the Road to Success

As time passed, Pfizer began to appreciate all Viagra could do, so they cloned it. As more and more men in the winters of their lives began to take it, it turned out that they needed less of the drug to get the same effect. Their blood levels were 40% higher than those under sixty-five. Then there were the guys with severe renal (kidney) insufficiency whose blood levels doubled if they took as much as men with mild or moderate renal disease. Drinkers who had developed cirrhosis had a 50% higher blood level on the same dose, because their 3A4 component was on permanent strike.

There were also some drugs that Viagra affected and some that had an impact on it. Alcohol and Amlodipine (Lotrel, Norvasc) were no problem, but Viagra's blood level was raised by:

- **Cimetidine (Tagamet)**
- **Erythromycin**
- **Ketoconazole (Nizoral)**
- **Itraconazole (Sporanox)**
- **Mibefradil (Posicor)**

These drugs rely on the same Cytochrome P450 system for metabolism. When Viagra has to compete with them to be first in line for cleavage, Viagra backs up in the body, and the overall blood level soars. Rifampin (Rifadin, Rifamate, Rifater) takes the wind out of Viagra's sails by lowering its overall level in the blood. Rifampin, a drug often used to treat TB, revs up the Cytochrome P450 system, a process known as enzyme induction.

Otherwise, Viagra kept to itself, leaving all other drugs alone.

After these early subjects, all of whom were believed to have psychological reasons for their erectile dysfunction, came eight double-blind, placebo-controlled crossover studies. Men with both psychological and organic reasons for their impotence were switched back and forth between Viagra and placebo, all the while recording the rigidity of their erections with penile plethysmography. Viagra's effects persisted for up to four hours in some lucky subjects but generally declined after two.

Side effects began to surface, many of them because Viagra can't keep from attacking PDE5 wherever it finds it:

- By dilating arteries in the brain, especially its protective outer lining, Viagra produced headaches in 16% of 734 patients
- Attacking vascular smooth muscle cells increased blood flow to the skin, producing

flushing and reddening of the face, neck
and/or trunk in 10% of Viagra takers
* Dyspepsia (an upset stomach that feels similar to heartburn) occurred in 7% due to
increased gastric blood flow
* Nasal congestion in 4%, diarrhea in 3%, and
dizziness in 2% of test subjects—all because
of Viagra's assaults on PDE5.

Then came the strange side effect. It turned out
that Viagra isn't so specific as to only affect PDE5
alone. Viagra likes PDE5 ten times more than it
likes PDE6, but it has a minor weakness for PDE6 as
well. PDE6 is found in the retina of the eye, where it
acts as an enzyme involved in the phototransduction
process that allows us to see colors. So it turns out
that when Viagra inhibits PDE6, about 3% of Viagra
takers feel as if they are looking at the world through
blue-tinted glasses. Some also lose the ability to tell
the difference between blue and green.

Most feel this is a small price to pay once they
understand that the strange side effect is harmless.
But since the drug has been released, ophthalmologists loath to have such a dramatic visual change
billed as harmless suggested that not enough long-term studies had been done to really say for sure that
the visual changes Viagra produce are harmless. The
long-term data on this question are still out.

Another side effect—the fact that 3% of patients
who took Viagra developed urinary tract infections—seems more likely to be related to the drug's
success at increasing the frequency of intercourse

than anything else. And almost any drug can give some people a rash, a kind of allergic reaction, as Viagra did with 2% of patients.

Like every drug that goes through the FDA approval process, Viagra has a long list of problems blamed on it as well, problems that occurred in under 2% of people who took it. Whether it caused these problems or not remains an open question, but Viagra adamantly states that there is "no improper relationship." To put these uncommon side effects in perspective, you may want to consult the *Physician's Desk Reference* and examine the host of uncommon reactions associated with aspirin. Because of the need to be certain that drugs are safe, such side effects are always reported even if there is no clear relationship between their occurrence and the medication itself.

MORE PATIENTS REPORT

For Jim, the twenty-eight-year-old MBA, the Viagra story was short but not sweet. He got it from a buddy who was passing them out in the office as a joke. He popped 50 mgs that night to see how it would work if he masturbated, anticipating using it on a date later in the week if it did. Viagra made Jim dizzy, made him see blue, and made him feel sick. Maybe, just maybe, it helped his erection be a little more rigid—but he wasn't sure. I wondered if maybe now we could settle down and start talking about his real problem: the ways he viewed himself as a man and the way he viewed and treated women. I wanted to see his identity delinked from his penile performance, linked to things he had a little more control over. Maybe his despair at the lack of an external fix-it for his psychological problems would spur a look inside instead.

Similarly, Bill and Janine, who had treated the advent of Viagra as the Second Coming that would save their troubled marriage, were disappointed at first. It turned out that Janine kept declining to try sex with Viagra as her fears about Bill's anger toward her and how that would be manifest in bed became clear. Rather than speak to him about her concerns, she would simply develop a headache on the way home from dinner. Bill was furious with her. After a couples session in which we discussed the underlying anger that was the real issue between them, we worked out a plan: The pair would negotiate three mutually acceptable dates. The first two would be preliminary, a time to talk about and plan their first night with the new pill before they actually tried it. They would specifically not attempt to have intercourse during these first two dates, though they could do everything else leading up to it. Then on the third date they would try to agree over dessert whether this was the right night to try Viagra. If it was, they would proceed. If not, they'd keep talking instead.

The results were much more impressive with this plan in place. The first two dates were the first time in a while that Bill and Janine had gotten a sitter and had a nice, quiet time together, talking over dinner without the looming question of whether there'd be sex and how Bill would function. The topics they discussed ranged from the phenomenon Viagra was becoming to their arguments over financial matters and the impact of these on their sex life. I had instructed them to think of three things they'd really liked about each other when they first met and discuss these as well, trying to guarantee for them some positive shared experiences over dinner.

Meanwhile, Bill was carrying the Viagra tablets his internist had given him around in his wallet like a talisman. Finally, the big night arrived. Bill, never one to want to be conservative where his manhood was concerned, took 100 mgs of Viagra after paying the check in the restaurant. The couple returned home and had sex. For Bill, the drug was a huge success. He felt better in bed than he had in a long time, his greater self-confidence also making him more gentle and more interested in Janine's response. But they were both disappointed that Janine wasn't well lubricated despite feeling excited, forcing them to resort to artificial lubricant. Janine was upset that she hadn't been able to come. Interestingly, though, because Bill was feeling more confident himself, he did more to stimulate her and was less put off by her inability to climax, less quick to conclude that it was her way to demonstrate another way in which he was not good enough.

Viagra was not a miracle cure for the long-standing relationship and sexual issues facing Bill and Janine. But it was not the neutron bomb I had feared, either. The availability of Viagra, combined with our interventions regarding how the couple relate to each other and continued couples therapy, will help Bill and Janine improve their marriage. It will also become more evident whether Viagra can indeed help women with erectile dysfunction as well. Perhaps it will help Bill and Janine with her problem achieving orgasm as well. Meanwhile, for the first time in years, they have a weekly date with each other that both consider inviolable: time to talk, time to relax, and time to make love. It may turn out that taking the time to be together emotionally and sexually that Viagra encourages is what really changes the lives of couples across America.

For Bob and Pete, though, it was the erections. Their life together was already rich and filled with love. Their relationship had endured for more years and across more crises than most anyone's I'd ever known. Pete's stellar reaction to 100 mgs seemed to signify to both men that he was alive and kicking. With all the muted competition and comparison that had gone on earlier about penises and even about the idea of impotence itself, I wasn't surprised to learn that Bob had Viagra envy. Just a quarter of one of Pete's tablets had Bob feeling like Matt Damon. Now that the issues about mortality and loss were more easily discussed between the pair, there was a palpable sense of relief and even levity between them. "Don't you up and die on me, you

old queen, now that you're better than ever in bed,"
Bob teased.

THE THREE TRIALS OF VIAGRA

Viagra was subjected to three sets of trials. The first
phase was informal and easy, twelve patients only.
The second phase, which established the incidence
of side effects and blood levels of the drug in
different groups of patients, was more arduous. But
with the third round of trials came the masses, lined
up around the block for a chance to see Viagra in
action. In the third round of twenty-one more ran-
domized double-blind, placebo-controlled trials of
up to six months' duration, men took fixed doses—
25, 50, or 100 mgs—of the drug or underwent a
careful titration of their dose.

Over three thousand patients aged nineteen to
eighty-seven years with erectile dysfunction of physiological (58%), psychological (17%), and mixed
physiological and psychological (24%) etiologies participated. The men were assessed with the International Index of Erectile Dysfunction at the beginning
and end of the treatment period. The researchers
convincingly confirmed what Fred had known years
before: Viagra helped men achieve erections suffi-
cient for sexual intercourse and improved their
ability to maintain erections after penetration. The
numbers got better as the dose got higher, with
success on both criteria in 63% of men on 25 mgs,

74% on 50 mgs, and 82% on 100 mgs (versus 24% of those with placebo reporting improvement in erections). In addition, 33% to 50% also reported successful intercourse at least once during a four-week treatment-free period.

While daily diaries showed no effect of medication on rates of attempted intercourse (twice weekly) there was clear treatment-related improvement in sexual functioning. Total successes divided by total attempts at intercourse were 66% on Viagra and 20% on placebo. These trials were generally three to six months long, with some patients continuing on Viagra for up to a year. Pfizer noted that few patients withdraw for any reason, including lack of effectiveness of the drug, while 88% reported Viagra had improved the frequency, firmness, and maintenance of erections; the frequency of orgasm; the frequency and level of desire; and the frequency, satisfaction, and enjoyment of intercourse. Not surprisingly, given all that, the overall level of relationship satisfaction was also improved.

Pfizer then showed that Viagra helped regardless of the baseline severity of erectile dysfunction as well as regardless of patient race, age, and the etiology of the erectile problem. Whether the impotence arose from coronary artery disease, hypertension, other cardiac or peripheral vascular disease, diabetes, depression, a radical prostatectomy or transurethral resection of prostate, a spinal cord injury, or cardiac and psychiatric medications didn't matter, though some groups had better responses than others.

About the only ones who couldn't take Viagra were those already on organic nitrites, including:

- Nitroglycerin (Nitro-bid, Nitrostat)
- Isosorbide Dinitrate (Isordil, Sorbitrate)
- Pentaerythritol Tetranitrate (Pentritol, Peritrate)
- Erythrityl Tetranitrate (Cardilate)

Viagra increased the drops in blood pressure already produced by these medications. Before the drug had been out a month, Pfizer experts were alerting gay activists to the dangers of Viagra and the perennially popular "poppers" taken in clubs. Poppers are inhaled and produce a "rush" that many people like. But because poppers are amyl nitrite, they can cause the same dramatic drops in blood pressure seen with nitrates used for cardiac conditions.

But after the trials, the company was compelled to proffer some other precautions as well, such as the fact that those with anatomical deformity of the penis (like that produced by Peyronie's disease—a hardened, fibrotic area on the penis that can cause curvature and pain with erection) or a condition known to produce priapism (sickle-cell anemia, multiple myeloma, leukemia) should use caution in using Viagra. Also, those with retinitis pigmentosa, a rare genetic disorder of phosphodiesterases, or other retinal problems such as macular degeneration should not take it or should keep the doses at the absolute lowest level possible.

Then came the "we don't knows," the disclaimers from Pfizer that said there were no studies of combination of Viagra with other drugs for erectile dysfunction. Although Viagra seemed safe with aspirin (150 mgs, the "baby" aspirin dose often used to prevent heart disease) in terms of bleeding time, it could theoretically cause bleeding because of its reaction with platelets in a test tube. Thus, there was also nothing known about its effects on bleeding in patients with peptic ulcers or bleeding disorders such as hemophilia.

Then came the phrases clearly added by attorneys: Pfizer delicately suggested that men should consider their level of cardiovascular health, given the physical exertion involved in intercourse. In other words, Pfizer did not intend to be liable for any rash of so-called coital coronaries that many anticipated in response to renewed sexual vigor in those whose cardiac arteries were as clogged as their penile ones. And, Pfizer gently reminded, Viagra provides no protection against sexually transmitted diseases such as hepatitis and AIDS—not to mention preventing pregnancy. Even a wonder drug has its limits.

Likewise, Pfizer sagely suggested that pregnant women not take Viagra despite the lack of mutagenicity, fertility impairment, teratogenicity, and embryotoxicity or fetotoxicity in rats, rabbits, and Chinese hamsters.

Even in men who took eight times the recommended highest dose (orgiastic overdosers), Viagra remained kind, merely causing somewhat more of the usual adverse events such as headaches, upset stomach, and flushing.

THE VIAGRA VERDICTS CONTINUE

Chris, supposedly eager to overcome his avoidance and lack of interest in sex, kept forgetting to make an appointment to see a urologist and get a prescription for Viagra. His girlfriend pressured him about it the same way she pressured him about what he was going to do after college and about how she fit into his plans. He became stubbornly determined, like a mule who sets himself in an oppositional stance and can't be budged. He attempted to draw me into the equation by asking me for a Viagra prescription, but I had already decided not to give the drug myself. If I pushed Viagra on Chris the way his girlfriend wanted to, I'd be acting intrusivly and controlling. I cared much more about understanding why Chris kept forgetting to make an appointment to get Viagra than about foisting it upon him. And I was particularly interested by the fact that as his girlfriend's unrelenting pressure continued, Chris's desire to expose himself mounted. I felt sure that the desire to avoid the disgust his girlfriend engendered during sex—and the adrenergic reaction that feeling engendered—was enough to defeat even the strongest of pills.

Meanwhile, Jane became the first woman I knew to try Viagra. Because her internist refused to prescribe it for women, she acquired it off the Internet under a false name for a fifty-dollar "doctor's fee" and the cost of the pills. She and I discussed the fact that this was an off-label use of the drug and that its efficacy and safety in women had not been adequately established. When the drug arrived, Jane's concerns about its safety quickly moved to the back burner, as she described being "wetter than ever" and finding vaginal intercourse more pleasurable than before. Her ability to reach orgasm, still somewhat delayed by Paxil, her antidepressant, was markedly improved as well. The last time I saw her, she was contemplating calling her boyfriend, Arthur, with whom she had since broken up, wondering if sex with him would be better now that she had Viagra on board. Whether she will and what will happen to their other relationship problems remains to be seen.

But my most favorite Viagra success story to date is Tom's. Just 25 mgs of Viagra worked like a charm for him. I could see the change in his erectile functioning projected in his demeanor and attitude. He took on the task of rehabilitation from his injury with renewed vigor and determination and started to say for the first time that he wanted to ride a bike again someday soon. As we explored his problems with his abandoning fiancée, Ellen, I could see him begin to understand that their relationship was built on a foundation of power struggles and issues about dominance and submission. So his feeling of being manipulated and dominated through her dramatic hissy fits was countered by his restraint of her during sex, perhaps the beginnings of sadomasochistic sexual fantasies of revenge. I hoped he would be able to find a relationship in which such struggles were not a necessary fuel for sex, since I had seen the many problems they ultimately engendered both within and outside the bedroom.

GET WITH THE PROGRAM

So Viagra, the once-lowly cardiac failure, had proven itself at last, risen to the top of the heap. It was discontinued less frequently due to side effects than a sugar pill. It was more sought after than the Spice Girls. At last there was an oral solution to the impotence problem that was highly effective, had few side effects, and was easily available with a simple, albeit expensive, prescription. (At the price of ten dollars per pill, one jaded Brooklyn subway rider complained that now he couldn't afford sex, either.)

But many men were ready to sell their boyhood baseball card collections, if need be, to procure Viagra. Unlike past treatments for impotence, there were no urethral applicators, no needles, no complicated devices, no surgeries to contend with. Once billed as the "Hottest New Drug Since Prozac," in its first month alone Viagra left that pill in the dust. But can Viagra give America the courage to change, to build a bridge to the twenty-first century's sexuality? Or is it merely the male equivalent of a Wonderbra, a technological trick to counter gravity, part of an ongoing quest to elude the effects of time? Everyone everywhere had an opinion. Everyone was getting with the program. Viagra became an overnight sensation.

7

Alternatives to Viagra

Not responding to Viagra may feel like the adult equivalent of not being chosen for the team. It may come as a blow to many men to find that they can't catch the wave, that their erectile dysfunction is too severe to be fixed by this miracle cure. But remember that if Viagra works in 70–80% of men depending on the cause of the erectile dysfunction, there are more than 20% it does not help. In certain groups such as those with nerve damage secondary to surgical procedures for prostate cancer, the number of success stories can even drop below 50%. So you're not alone if the wonder drug of the nineties passes you by. There are even websites where men who didn't respond to Viagra can commiserate, if you need to chat.

This chapter will take a look at how treatments for erectile dysfunction evolved, swooping into the patent office to revisit some strange inventions that were supposed to help. It will also discuss how to regroup and what to try next if Viagra has let you down: the pros and cons of the alternatives, as well as the costs and dose regimens generally prescribed.

And we'll look ahead to see what other oral impotence treatments are in the pipeline.

ALTERNATIVES FROM THE EARLY DAYS

One early alternative to cure impotence dates back five thousand years but also remains popular today: Yohimbine is the active ingredient that's extracted from the bark of the African yohimbe tree. It seems to work by stimulating pleasure centers in the brain and boosting libido. In addition, it causes small blood vessel dilation, which leads to a more forceful erection, not unlike Viagra.

Many men claim yohimbine increases orgasmic pleasure as well, which is not surprising given its effects on dopamine and norepinephrine, the same brain chemicals affected by antidepressants such as Buproprion (Wellbutrin) and Venlafaxine (Effexor). Like those mind-altering, mood-elevating substances, yohimbine must be taken for about three to four weeks before it works. In a recent study, even rats liked it, with those receiving the substance engaging in twice as much sex as rats that didn't get it, creating a sort of Rat Pack Baby Boom. It has shown no serious side effects so far despite centuries of use.

A second popular remedy for erectile dysfunction is red ginseng, an herb popular in China which has been shown to improve erectile rigidity as well as heighten libido and increase sexual pleasure. Since ginseng literally means "man root" and looks amusingly similar to the human phallus, it's not surprising that somewhere along the way someone suspected it was an aphrodisiac or an aid to potency as well. Like yohimbine it is safe and has few side effects. However, a recent report suggested that many of the vials of ginseng available in convenience stores around the country are largely alcohol. This suggests that if you want to try ginseng you should obtain it from a reliable health food store and read package labels carefully.

Other once-popular remedies such as the highly toxic Spanish Fly and various animal organs have no known medicinal value. The fact that they're of no benefit hasn't stopped poachers from seeking the genitals of large and ferocious animals ranging from tigers to rhinos. These and other impotence remedies seem to have little demonstrable medicinal value, but given what we know about the role of flagging self-confidence and anxiety in erectile dysfunction, it is not surprising that a placebo (sugar pill) effect would occur in men with erectile dysfunction.

THE ADVENT OF HYDRAULIC DEVICES

After turning away from nature in search of potency potions, man turned to his own ingenuity in designing machines that pump up his penis. The first sex patent in the U.S. was granted to Dr. John Beers of Rochester, N.Y., in 1846 for his "Wife's Protector," a kind of vaginal diaphragm used for contraception with a shape that seems based on the good doctor's equipment for working with teeth. We can only speculate about how many penises rebelled when confronted with entering a vagina wired with dental works. Talk about vagina dentata!

Then came the Victorian era, when most patents for both men and women were designed to control masturbation, the solitary vice believed to lead to hairy palms, blindness and general mental degeneracy of the type described in great and graphic detail in von Krafft-Ebbing's epic work "Psychopathia Sexualis." Next was the assault on wet dreams, which many held were the nighttime expression of degenerate daytime thoughts. The new penile rings pierced the penis at night if the poor plebe wearing one got an erection. The Victorians had their own anti-emission laws.

The prevailing view of erectile dysfunction was that men who suffered from it had used up their sexual energy in some perverted and onanistic way such as masturbation or nocturnal emission. Thus, it was their fault if they were now ill-equipped for normal adult sexuality. With the discovery of electricity came new hope as some desperate erectile dysfunction sufferers purchased electrified jock straps from mail order catalogues.

Then came a kind of Victorian crackdown in America as Charles Goodyear proffered the world's first vulcanized rubber, whose role as a protective barrier that could prevent pregnancy was quickly grasped. A new sexual revolution was summarily stalled by killjoy Anthony Comstock, who believed that premarital sex and contraception were both ungodly. He fought for the passage of the Comstock Law, which was in effect from 1873 through the 1920s. This law prohibited the distribution of rubbers and other articles used for immoral purposes such as enjoying sex. As luck would have it, rubber turned out to be essential and widely used for combating impotence even though it was banned from use in condoms for many years. Many men, including Dr. James Dunn, began recommending it to trap blood in the unwilling corpuses of men who suffered from erectile problems. Essentially, a rubber band could be secured around the base of the penis to keep whatever erection a man could obtain in place by blocking the outflow of blood. Patents for penile dorsal vein clamps quickly followed. These devices were all variations on the rubber band at the base of the penis, and occluded the flow of blood out of the penis, much like a stopper in a bathtub. However, all these devices could kill the cavernosal smooth muscle cells if left on for too long (more than thirty minutes), making the problem worse.

The first pneumatic or pump devices were invented around 1917, when Otto Lederer received a patent for a rubber chamber that fit entirely over the penis. A pressure bulb at the top created negative pressure and drew blood into the penis while a band around the base kept it there. Surprisingly, given their effectiveness, it was sixty-six years before they were mass marketed. Better plastics and a more liberal social milieu came together in the sixties and seventies as men such as Marvin Burdette and Geddings Osbon made penile pumps for their own use. Osbon marketed his under the name Erecaid after being granted a patent in 1983.

Penile pumps are straightforward and highly successful if cumbersome to use: A plastic cylinder is placed over the penis, and air is drawn out of it through some sort of pump, creating negative pressure on the penis and producing an influx of blood in a simple hydraulic manner. After several minutes of pumping, a flexible ring reminiscent of erector rings is placed around the penis and an erection occurs. Despite the popularity of rubber bands earlier on, regular rubber bands are not recommended. Pumps are safe, generally always successful if used correctly, relatively side-effect free and can be used as often as desired, provided individual erections are maintained for less than thirty minutes to prevent damage to the delicate cavernosal smooth muscle cells. On the downside, pumps can produce discolored, cold and misshapen penises in long-time users as well as mild discomfort on ejaculation due to the constriction of the urethral channel produced by the ring around the base of the penis. This can put a definite damper on that moment of airborne excitement that orgasm should be.

Users also complain about the lack of spontaneity involved in interrupting lovemaking to pump. Some men also claim their erections are wobbly at the base and not as rigid as they want. Though they have undergone limited testing, one study reported a success rate of about 90%, higher than Viagra. Pumps remain a viable and safe alternative for those for whom Viagra just doesn't work or has intolerable side effects. The pump can be dangerous in patients with blood disorders that make the blood more prone to clot, stickier or thicker than usual (such as sickle cell anemia) or those who bleed easily (such as hemophiliacs). A survey of 5,847 vacuum users showed that 83.5% continued to use the device over time and were happy with its desired effects as well as its side effects. The pump costs anywhere from $300 to $600, with variable insurance reimbursement.

In the mid-1960s, while the pump was being perfected in the bedrooms of its adventuresome inventors, the concept of penile implants was being developed. There are two types of penile implants:

The non-hydraulic kind consists of placing a pair of semi-rigid, malleable silicone rods into the corpus cavernosum. These rods create a permanent erection that can be bent down alongside the body when not desired, then easily and swiftly bent up into place to allow a functional erection for intercourse when warranted. Because these devices make the penis longer than it would be otherwise, they can either inspire envy in others or evoke embarrassment for the owner in the urinal.

The hydraulic inflatable penile implant involves the placement of two extremely thin cylinders alongside the corpus cavernosum with a pumping mechanism placed inside the scrotum. When this pump is squeezed a few times, a small pouch placed in the abdomen sends saline solution to the inflatable cylinders. Like water balloons, these cylinders then expand and grow rigid, mimicking the normal erection process. Pushing a valve at the top of the pump after intercourse releases the erection, and the saline returns to its abdominal chamber. Newer hydraulic models can even contain all the necessary parts within the penis itself, meaning that when you want an erection you simply bend or squeeze the head of the penis.

With these implants, the penis is soft under normal circumstances but offers predictable erections on demand with no shots, pumps or sex therapy. Expensive to the tune of $15,000, these implants are covered by most insurance plans. But beware: They are irreversible and actually damage the erectile tissue of the penis further. So don't expect to take them out and try Viagra later. Implant surgery takes one to three hours and may have to be repeated if the implant gets infected or malfunctions. Even if all goes well, you can expect your erections to be less long and less thick than before but still adequate for intercourse.

Despite these drawbacks (and unlike the vacuum pump, penile injections and suppositories and even Viagra) both types of implants allow instant erections. The implant option may still be the best for men with severe erectile dysfunction that Viagra doesn't help. However, although studies have shown these devices are technically satisfactory in 75–90% of cases, the satisfaction of the men's partners generally does not match the seeming technical success of the surgery.

Vascular surgery began in about 1973, the dawn of the age of other arterial unclogging procedures such as those used in angioplasty today to get all that leftover sludge out of those coronary arteries. Most vascular surgery is aimed at repairing injured arteries or clearing them of blockages. When it works, it can restore erectile function to a great extent—when it works. The initial success rates were quite low but have improved, with better ways to sort out who will really benefit from surgery.

One interesting method of vascular surgery is to flip the deep dorsal vein around and connect it with the artery above the problem area, in effect changing the vein to an artery. Since the veins are much less muscular and more easily distended than the adamant arteries, these reversed veins can carry a good amount of blood into the corpus cavernosum, promoting erections. Another possibility is to use microsurgery to promote re-vascularization of the penis. However, vascular surgery is only appropriate for highly selected cases, with only about 7% of men with impotence eligible. The success, when the surgery is applied to appropriate candidates, is permanent and approaches 70%. It works best on young men whose blood flow problems stem from trauma such as accidents that damage the penis.

The age of injectable impotence treatments was ushered in by the shot heard round the world: Surgeon Ronald Virag's inadvertent injection of papaverine into the penis of his anesthetized patient, who promptly spiked a lengthy erection. At the same time, another injectable, phenoxybenzamine, was being used to produce erections, but it caused patients to feel nauseated, hyperventilate and have heart arrhythmias. Continuing a long tradition of physicians who experiment on themselves, fifty-seven-year-old British physician Giles Brindley stepped out from behind a lectern in 1983 and dropped his britches to expose his erect, self-injected phallus, injected with phenoxybenzamine. Then there was the equally devoted if more subdued Adrian Zorgniotti, one of the first to use papaverine and phentolamine (Regitine) injections and the first to give patients phentolamine tablets of his own design, later impregnating a strip of paper with the liquid drug which worked within twenty minutes when held between the cheek and gum.

Injectable prostaglandin E-1 (PGE1, a.k.a. alprostadil) followed and soon a combination of these three drugs (papaverine, phentolamine, and prostaglandin E-1) became the norm. The initial use of papaverine alone had caused prolonged erections as well as the fibrosis or scarring of the corpus callosum, which you can guess is bad for erectile functioning in the long term. The tri-mix allowed the overall dose of papaverine to be reduced to about 10% of the amount needed when it was used alone. Specifically designed and custom-made phentolamine pills became the first oral treatment ever, but some of the patients who took them fainted, a definite impediment to lovemaking.

All of these potions were initially designer drugs, made especially for patients by physicians or pharmacists in specific and expensive batches.

It was not until 1995 that Caverject (PGE1, alprostadil) hit the mass market in injectable form. When injected into the base of the penis it relaxed smooth muscles, promoting erections through vasodilation. Though effective in over 50% of patients, many found the option of self-injection made them squeamish, and it was a painful beginning to the lovemaking process. The pain was intensified by the inflammatory effects of the prostaglandin on the delicate cavernosal tissue, which meant it couldn't be used daily. Still, for many men Caverject was far less painful than the bruised egos accompanying impotence.

Caverject heralded the onset of the woody-while-mowing-the-lawn era, since sexual stimulation was irrelevant for the drug to take action. When injected it reliably produced erections in fifteen to thirty minutes that lasted up to an hour, even in the absence of desire. There were attempts to make the injections more palatable, with one well-known and usually on-the-mark sex therapist advising, "Injecting yourself can interfere with spontaneity, but this is easily remedied by making the shot a part of loveplay."

Still, at twenty dollars a shot, Caverject was the first nonmechanical, nonsurgical, widely available means of treating impotence. It boosted the sales of erectogenic solutions from practically nothing to 6.4 million dollars in 1995. It was a sign of things to come.

By 1997 the cheaper and less painful Edex was out, still PDE1 (alprostadil) but with a slightly different formulation than Caverject, which made it possible to use a smaller needle. Like Caverject, it is injected ten minutes to two hours before sex and also gives erections lasting more than one hour, often even after ejaculation.

Still awaiting release is Invicorp, a mix of a protein called VIP and phentolamine, which also dilates smooth muscle cells more effectively and with less pain than alprostadil. Still, it seems likely that the VIPs behind this drug's development are feeling the pain as Viagra rises. After all, a major advance of their drug was to be the fact that it was taken just before sex and required stimulation to produce an erection rather than the automatic, mowing-the-lawn erections of the others. But Invicorp is injectable while Viagra, which also requires user stimulation to work, is oral. The future for injectable treatments was pretty much killed with the advent of Viagra, except for those men in whom local delivery of the drug was more beneficial than a systemic oral medication.

Though you'd think it was self-evident, a study was actually done to find out why men dropped out of treatment with injectable agents. In a group of 180 men averaging fifty-eight years old, 22% quit after a test injection with papaverine/phentolamine or PGE1. Over half dropped out by the end of a year and only 20% were satisfied. Almost 8% noted disappearance of their symptoms when confronted with the injections, raising the question of whether it is indeed possible to be scared stiff. Interestingly, over 57% of those who quit cited loss of interest in sex as the reason, while another 15% chose the vacuum pump or an implant instead. Patients with psychogenic etiologies for their erectile difficulties were the most satisfied with the injection therapies, perhaps because they also work in the absence of desire, a truly totally automatic point-and-shoot cycle that your mind can't mess with.

Of those who took the shots for five years, 94% reported being satisfied with the results with only 7% having had prolonged erections and only 3% reporting penile nodules at the injection site.

As an aside, though, these prolonged erections are a genuine urological emergency regardless of what produces them. The lack of oxygen caused by overly long blood pooling in the penis causes intense pain. The cure for priapism is—guess what—putting a needle into the corpus cavernosum to draw off part of the blood it contains. Or the injection of a sympathetic nervous system medication that immediately shuts down the parasympathetic nervous system tone in the region and lulls your penis into relaxing. Priapism (named for Priapus, the Greek god of procreation) is also caused by the antidepressant agent Trazadone (Deseryl). This medication is used primarily in women because it can produce priapism in men. Priapism produced by any means—Trazadone, oral agents like Viagra, injections, or mechanical restriction of blood flow caused by bands around the penis—is an emergency because it kills those precious smooth muscle cavernosal cells.

If the VIPs at Invicorp are envious of Viagra, it's also safe to say that the folks at Vivus, who just released MUSE in 1997, are anything but amused. The first alprostadil administered in pellet form, MUSE is inserted into the urethra with a tiny plastic applicator resembling a plunger, which must be placed about an inch and a half into the tender opening of the urethra. Though you can use the drug twice a day, it's not recommended that you do if your partner is pregnant. MUSE can be used five to ten minutes before sex and results in an automatic erection lasting up to an hour.

Even less humorous to the MUSE folks is the fact that they paved the way for Viagra, with MUSE sending potency drug sales rocketing to about $150 million in 1997 and prescriptions to over 600,000 men in the first year alone. Vivus is now scrambling to try to figure out how to revive itself: As of April 6, 1998, they increased their sales force from 74 to 280 and started a counterattack, arguing that MUSE works locally whereas Viagra invades the entire body. They tried to play up the side effects that Viagra's systemic invasion causes, but by then the entire country had gotten Viagra under its skin.

If Viagra didn't work for you and these earlier options seem unappealing, hang on. Even as Viagra skyrockets, there are starstruck understudies waiting in the wings. Vasomax, the oral form of phentolamine, is marketed by an upstart biotech company called Zonagen, whose stock went up despite the fact that the product wasn't so effective. It blocks adrenaline and relaxes smooth muscle tissue, dilating arteries. Zonagen says it helped 60-80% of those tested, with fewer side effects than Viagra, the main one being a stuffy nose. It can be taken as little as twenty to forty minutes before sex, requiring stimulation to work. But the FDA was unconvinced by the data and requested that more studies be done, sending Zonagen stock into a tailspin and causing some to speculate about whether the drug will ever actually make it to the market at all.

Spontane (apomorphine) is a central nervous system stimulator in the morphine family that triggers brain centers involved in sexual response. In FDA trials at the moment, it seems to be working in about

70% of patients. Since its mechanism of action is different from Viagra's, it may be a good alternative for those who don't respond. Still, Spontane's membership in the morphine family may hamper its marketability. Though it's true that it isn't addictive, getting people to believe that will be difficult.

So for now, and probably for some time to come, Viagra is king. No mere fifteen minutes of fame for Pfizer. By May 5, 1998, it was accounting for nineteen out of twenty new impotence prescriptions. Some projected first year sales of up to $10 billion worldwide. The early numbers showed that Viagra was prescribed to 36,700 men in week one, 115,000 in week two and 208,000 in week three of its entry onto the market, triple the rate of Prozac in its youth.

Pulling the covers off impotence the way Prozac demystified depression, Viagra may have opened up new possibilities even if it hasn't worked for you. If you were one of the more than 95% of men with erectile dysfunction who didn't seek treatment before Viagra's release, you may now know more about your penis and its problems than ever. You may feel that it is more acceptable to broach the subject with your doctor. So even if Viagra doesn't work for you, you may be ready to try an alternative to it. Your days of taking the problem lying down may be behind you. As you've seen, some of the other treatments outlined may even have advantages over Viagra, such as not requiring ingestion of a chemical, acting locally, or working for more severe cases of impotence.

Still, it's not surprising that you'd be singing a different kind of Viagra blues than all those men who are looking at the world through rose-colored (if blue-tinted) glasses right now. Even if you're not overtly depressed by your lack of a Viagra Victory, seeing a psychiatrist or therapist may be another good alternative to Viagra for some people. The next chapter will look at what individual psychotherapy, couples therapy and sex therapy have to offer instead of—or in addition to—Viagra or other medications.

8

How Talking Can Help

Although the penile apparatus used in achieving erection is complicated, it's nothing compared to all those billions and billions of interconnected nerve cells that make up your mind. That three pounds of pudding you carry around between your ears can certainly cause lots of trouble when it comes to sex.

The actual steps of the sexual response cycle, especially desire, are immensely influenced by the construction of your core sexual identity. Sex with a partner calls into play all the aspects of both of your sexual identities as well as the ways in which you relate to others. And as we saw with Janine and Bill, a little bit of intervention in therapy can go quite a long way. Imagine what would have happened if Bill had insisted on taking Viagra when and where he wanted and made matters worse by angrily forcing himself on Janine. Or imagine the result if Janine had failed to understand how her concerns—and anger—about Bill's dominance represented by the pill were making her less interested in being sexual with Bill.

When are sexual problems, including erectile dysfunction, worth talking about with a professional? Simply put, it's when you feel that your innermost thoughts and feelings, your behaviors or your interactions with your partner are a problem. If you have feelings and fantasies that stir up uncomfortable emotions, talking about them may help. If you're plagued by certain behaviors that seem out of your control (e.g., compulsive masturbation), if your unwillingness or inability to engage in certain behaviors (e.g., oral sex) is causing you or your partner distress, talking may help. And, of course, if you desire to do something that's considered criminal, like Chris's desires to expose himself, you should seek therapy to understand more about why. Finally there's the flexibility factor: if you always need certain things to get aroused or you can never do certain things in bed, your sexual range—and your enjoyment of your sexual self—is constricted. Psychotherapy can help you to become more flexible, which is usually accompanied by having more fun in the sack.

There are several kinds of therapies that can be useful for patients with erectile dysfunction. It will take a trained professional to help you understand which is right for you and why. In what follows, I'll review the various kinds of sexual issues I encounter in individuals and couples and explore what types of treatment are usually effective.

EXPLORING INNER CONFLICTS

Your core sexual identity is made up of your gender identity and comfort with whatever gender role you've adopted, your sexual orientation, and your sexual intention—what you'd like to do sexually and with whom. These components then influence your sexual responses, from desire to arousal to orgasm.

Although your core sexual identity is reflected in your behaviors during sex, notice that all the elements of that identity are represented in your head—in your fantasy life—first. You have to fantasize about cross-dressing before you can actually do it. You won't just wake up one day and find yourself in silk stockings. It's important to realize that most fantasies are laden with conflict. They have two sides to them and they are used to manage our anxiety and protect us from feeling overwhelmed. So fantasizing about being the opposite gender can be a way of relieving ourselves from the burdens of being a man for the moment, having to perform in whatever ways we think a man should perform. Sexual thoughts, feelings and behaviors, like all thoughts, feelings and behaviors, always have two sides to them. What we think, feel and do is a product of those two sides competing to find the balance that will make us most comfortable.

Fantasies give us hints about who we really are, which can stir up anxiety. Because of this some people deal with fantasies by total repression and disavowal. But repressed fantasies tend to break out of the cages we've created for them at inopportune moments. Keeping them under wraps can be a full time job which can make us feel dull and empty sexually. Psychotherapy can provide a safe place where you can begin to explore both sides of your fantasies and the feelings they engender. This usually involves teaching people to see that their fantasies are often not the huge cinematic releases they seem to expect but fleeting images, fragments of stories. Exploring these and learning how to embroider on them with less anxiety in therapy can open up new avenues to understanding yourself sexually.

JOHN

When we first started working together to address his potency problems, John denied that he had any fantasies. His impotence evaluation had been negative and there was no reason to suspect organic causes for his problems. He denied having not only sexual fantasies, but fantasies in general, such as where his career might be in five years. Over time he started to notice that he had fleeting images of being tied up when he masturbated, and he admitted that he would sometimes tweak his nipple extra hard or be rough in how he touched his penis. He found this embarrassing to talk about but pleasurable to do.

When I inquired as to whether there was a partner he imagined doing these things to him, he blushed before confessing he had intermittent images of a cold, Nordic, Sharon Stone type in mind who teased him in bed. I had the sense that he wouldn't fully let himself see any more than her outlines, wouldn't flesh her out in his mind. He was playing a kind of psychic peek-a-boo with the object of his desire. It turned out that this Sharon Stone character reminded him of an old girlfriend who used to growl at him playfully during sex and threaten him with her long, catlike nails. She could provoke waves of pleasure by running them down his chest and along his inner thighs, perilously close to his genitals. He had found this immensely erotic. Remembering the image of this girlfriend made him suddenly recall his actual role in their game together: that of lion-tamer.

Through psychotherapy, John came to see that he did indeed want to tame the women he fantasized about. In fact, he became increasingly aware of the fantasy of whipping them into submission, of dominating them through rape. To be sure he was kept under control and didn't really enact his forbidden sadistic desires, he had performed a complicated series of psychological somersaults. First, he'd switched places, made Sharon Stone the aggressor. Then he'd distanced himself from acknowledging the fantasy itself, and he removed the historical reference in his memory to his former girlfriend and what she did that turned him on. By denying he even had fantasies, he'd protected himself from his feelings of guilt about his sadistic urges. Nevertheless, an awareness of his aggressive urges sneaked through, and produced his symptom of impotence. John's impotence was the result of anxiety, some sense of danger that the carefully hidden fantasy might emerge and overwhelm him. It was also an expression of the other side of the conflict: John's wishes to be loving and close, not to hurt his partner, to risk being hurt himself rather than hurting her. It's harder to rape a partner, pound her into submission, when you can't get an erection. The loss of the erection was in a way an expression of love and a desire not to hurt. But the sense that his partner had somehow made him lose his masculinity also intensified John's desires to dominate her, creating a vicious cycle that increased the anxiety he felt and furthered his erectile dysfunction.

The problems we have trying to manage and balance our competing wishes, fantasies, and fears can be profitably talked about in psychotherapy, helping to produce an improved understanding of whom we are, what our sexual identity is. Psychotherapy can help us see the flip side of the conflicts that drive fantasy and behavior. It can also help understand the sources of the anxiety, anger, shame, disgust and discomfort they sometimes engender. Sometimes understanding the underlying conflict will make your sexual interest in a certain fantasy or behavior decline. Other times it will free you up to enjoy the imagery of the fantasy with less guilt, to recognize that your thoughts can't really hurt anyone. Still other times it will enable you to weigh the costs and benefits of actually enacting it. Our inner fantasies that contribute to our core sexual identities are a veritable internal circus taking place under the Big Top that is our skull. Learning to be a more effective ringmaster often involves gaining an indepth knowledge of all the acts and a sense of comfort with them. Then you can sit back, relax and enjoy the show. Much of the problem surrounding fantasy is that too often we act as if thinking the thought is the same as doing the deed. If you think about having sex with another woman when you're with your wife, is that a problem? If you think that the thought itself is the same as having really cheated on her, it will be. Many religions such as Catholicism treat the thought and the deed as identical to each other. That means if you give free reign to the full range of inner fantasies you have you can end up feeling pretty guilty. If you insist on holding this view of things, what you actually consider acceptable to think about can become enormously constricted, to the detriment of your sexual functioning and identity. You will find you have put the very things that could spice up your sex life off limits to your mind.

Guilt makes people confess. So if you have fantasies about someone else while sleeping with your wife and you feel guilty about it, you just may tell her, hurting her feelings and creating all the ingredients for a huge blow-up. If you understood better the distinction between thought and deed, you would feel less guilty and have less need to confess. Having access to your inner fantasies can allow you to indulge them more readily, which in turn can promote a stronger sense of desire and arousal. You can actually take the images and play around with them, evoke them as a means of heightening your interest and pleasure both during sex and even when just fantasizing about it. That image of sex with another woman may actually make things spicier with your wife—but only if you aren't feeling like a guilty adulterer. Guilt, shame and anxiety can zap your erectile functioning.

Even when we do know what we want and we express our fantasies in behavior, they can still conjure up feelings of guilt, shame and anxiety. Once we actually behave in a particular way with a partner, we may spend our time feeling concerned about what our actions transmit about us and worrying about what our partner is thinking. These negative feelings come about because our wants and our desires are not one-sided but conflict-laden. They usually revolve around whom the other person represents to us: a siren, causing us to crash against the rocks? Mother, scolding us for touching ourselves "down there'? Most likely it is a blend of people to be sorted out and understood. To really understand our sexual fantasies and feelings we also need to have an understanding of how we approach relationships, what we think they revolve around and who our sexual partners remind us of or represent from our pasts.

This type of treatment is geared toward helping you increase your awareness and appreciation of your core sexual identity, understanding and accepting its conflict-laden nature and coming to believe in your heart that thoughts are not the same as deeds. In this way you gain the fullest access possible to the various parts of yourself, the lion tamer as well as the lion. Gaining this type of understanding can be time consuming and expensive. It involves exploring early-life relationships that shaped your fantasies as well as the details of your inner world. It is, in effect, the Rolls Royce of engine repairs, like taking your sexual motor apart, examining all the pieces and reassembling them so that they run better, making nips and tucks and adding new parts when necessary.

CHANGING PROBLEMATIC THOUGHTS AND BEHAVIORS

There's also room for a simple visit to Jiffy Lube to get you back on the road to feeling good sexually. Another less intensive level at which therapeutic intervention can be pitched is that of problematic patterns of thought and behaviors. These cognitive-behavioral techniques do not attempt to uncover how your patterns of thinking and behaving came to be as they are. Instead, they take those patterns themselves as a starting point and work to change them.

THINKING DIFFERENTLY

We discussed the fact that men with erectile dysfunction often have extremely critical thoughts about themselves after they fail to get and keep an erection. Intervening cognitively might involve getting a man to write down and challenge all those pejorative self-evaluations. For example, if Tim thinks, "I'm a real wimp, a sissy" when he fails to get an erection, a cognitive behavioral therapist might ask him to write down that thought and then argue with himself about it. "I'm not really a wimp, I just had a problem this one time. But I'm working on it. And a sissy would be someone who couldn't face it, which is not me." Rather than allowing yourself to wallow in negative thoughts, a patient in this kind of treatment will challenge them at every turn, arguing himself out of the notion that he is a sissy.

Another kind of cognitive modification that can help your sexual functioning involves an examination of what kinds of causal attributions you make about your erectile difficulties. Let's say that you didn't get an erection the last time you attempted sex. Joe might explain the problem to himself by saying that he was tired or that he feels that his partner's perfume was too strong and he found it unappealing. Joe might write off the erectile problem as a one-time thing. Brad, on the other hand, might question his entire manhood, feel the problem will never go away and personalize it, blaming himself.

In sexual functioning, as in life more generally, people who explain bad events such as impotence to themselves as specific ("I was tired"), temporary ("It's a one-time thing") and external ("Her perfume was a turnoff") are more optimistic about their future prospects for success. Those who explain bad events globally ("I'm a wimp"), permanently ("It'll never change") or internally ("It's my fault") are more pessimistic.

The set of attributional qualities in response to good events (i.e., getting and keeping a good erection) is the opposite for optimists and pessimists: The sexual optimist sees good events as a reflection of global, permanent and internal factors. He says, "I've always generally been a good lover." The pessimist sees good events as specific, fleeting and external: "I got lucky this one time because she was really hot in bed and handled my penis just right."

While these cognitions are driven by our views of our core sexual identities, our self-esteem, and our history of how we relate to others, changing them doesn't always need to involve delving into these thoughts and feelings in depth as in an exploratory treatment. The act of challenging and attempting to restructure thinking alone can often be enough to make a difference in how men think, feel, and act during sex. Of course, there can be a downside to the externalization that makes us sexually optimistic: It can cause us to fail to take responsibility for things that really are our fault. Nevertheless, it may be worth trying to shift your thinking if it promotes better sexual functioning.

BEHAVING DIFFERENTLY

Other psychological treatments focus in on behavior itself, bypassing thoughts, feelings, and fantasies and addressing what someone is actually doing. Behavioral treatments for erectile dysfunction involve interventions geared to get men to act differently in how they approach sex. For example, there are so-called sensate focus exercises in which a man is asked to focus in on the sensations aroused in his penis by touching it or having a partner touch it when it is soft. The goal here is to focus on how it feels without regard to whether it gets erect or not. In fact, in some exercises, getting an erection is grounds for stopping the exercise and waiting until the erection wanes. The focus is on sensation, not stiffness or performance success.

Another behavioral exercise might involve getting and losing an erection over and over again during masturbation, until the feeling of a waning erection does not inspire the sense of panic that it once did. This is a form of systematic desensitization, the unlinking of erectile dysfunction and anxiety.

These behavioral techniques have much in common with the practices of Tantric yoga and massage, a spiritual system of sexuality that originated in Tibet. In Tantric sex, the focus is on stimulation without ejaculation, which results in long sessions of lovemaking that are said to have spiritual benefits as well.

Like cognitive therapy, behavioral therapy does not focus on where the problematic behavior comes from internally. It does not address those problems of sexual identity that lead to problems with desire, arousal and orgasm. It focuses instead on changing how you behave. The same behavioral pattern (problems getting an erection, for example) can come from many different sources. Sometimes just trying to alter the behavior without tracking it back to those sources within the individual is adequate. When it is, it's cheaper, easier and there's nothing wrong with it. But often a more intensive, inner-directed approach is still needed. The psychodynamic approach can provide a safe setting for exploring where your mind goes when you let it before looking at how your innermost desires are transformed into thoughts and actions.

COUPLES THERAPY

All of the approaches described above, from psychodynamic to cognitive to behavioral, can also be conducted with couples as well as individuals. A qualified therapist can help a couple investigate their individual thoughts and feelings and how these fit or don't fit together. If you've got a man with a desire for domination and rape and a woman who is aroused by that loss of control, there may be no problem (unless the fantasies are a cover for acting out other hostilities and problems in the relationship). But if you have all sorts of negative feelings and fantasies about oral sex and your partner requires it to feel fulfilled, then there may be an issue to contend with.

Similarly, problematic patterns of thinking are often evident in couples and follow the same patterns you might expect based on what I told you about the explanations we give ourselves. If a man sees a problem between him and his wife as global ("She hates sex"), permanent ("She always has and always will"), or maliciously motivated ("She refuses to have sex, just to annoy me"), there's probably going to be a great deal of tension within the couple. But if he sees it as specific, temporary, and unmotivated ("She didn't like oral sex this one time, but she seemed like she was trying it anyway"), there's less anger and more of a chance to work things out, more hopefulness that they will change in the future.

Behavioral approaches such as sensate focus exercises (focusing on sensation rather than performance) and systematic desensitization (the stopping and starting that de-links erectile dysfunction and panic) can also be done between partners as well as alone, especially after the partner with erectile dysfunction has mastered them during masturbation.

Probably the most important role of couples therapy is to repair and improve damaged communication between partners that can either arise from or contribute to erectile dysfunction. There are several ways in which communication goes astray between two people.

REPAIRING BROKEN PHONE LINES

First, there's the well-documented fact that men and women, on average, communicate differently. To women, talking means discussing feelings and personal reactions. To men it often involves what linguist Deborah Tannen has dubbed "report talk," the kind of conversation in which a man explains events to a woman, saying "We had a meeting at work" when what she's really wanting to know is "How did you feel about how it went." Her attempts to get this information out of her reluctant partner may make him feel intruded upon, or he may have more distance from his feelings than she does, the result of the pressures to minimize and conceal them that many men have experienced in childhood.

These basic communication problems are often magnified when couples try to talk about sex, which is a sensitive issue that evokes strong reactions. A couples therapist can help couples communicate better about this difficult topic. The saying that all's fair in love and war may be true, but if you engage in communication within your relationship as if it were war, casualties are the result. Among the common weapons of mate destruction couples therapist Bernie Zilbergeld observes are:

- Attack and defend: "You did x." "I did not."
- Monstrifying your partner: "You're a whining bitch who's out to destroy me."
- Sulk and destroy: Withdrawing and refusing to talk, the silent treatment
- Finding allies: "Well, my therapist thinks you're a schmuck, too!"
- Going for the jugular: Knowing your partner's vulnerabilities and moving in on them

The first thing a good couples therapist will do is to call a temporary truce, a cease fire of sorts. The next thing will be to begin, as I did with Bill and Janine, to try to structure their time together so that it includes adequate time to talk, to be together and to play. There are often limits set by the therapist on what can be talked about, so that some topics that are especially volatile are saved for sessions, when the therapist can act as referee and challenge the problematic patterns of communication.

One of the main things I believe people typically do when they fail to communicate is to make inferences about what their partner is thinking and feeling. Good communication means focusing on telling your partner what you think and feel as tactfully, clearly, and directly as possible, without accusation. Since you cannot know for sure what your partner is thinking and feeling unless he or she tells you, you need to help provide a safe environment in which to do the same thing. Then at most you can rephrase your best understanding of what your partner is saying to see if you've got it right.

Another thing couples tend to do wrong is to make value judgments about differences. The partner whose sex drive is higher may judge his mate to be abnormally disinterested. That's not a good place to start from in trying to understand what each of you wants and strike a compromise. Many couples have their most intense talks when they are angry, so the chances that they will focus on what's right instead of wrong with the relationship and on what they like as well as what they need to change or work on is practically nil. Fighting while angry also tips the scales in favor of making the global, permanent, blaming attributions about a problem that will make your partner's blood boil and reduce your chances of reaching agreement.

Once couples have reached a truce as well as gained some of the skills needed to communicate better, the next task of couples therapy is usually to try to ascertain what both partners need and want, what turns them on in bed. This will often highlight the ways in which they are different and set the stage for negotiations to begin about what steps can be taken to give each partner the most of what she wants and needs. If this step goes well, couples are back on the same side again, ready to begin to make creative compromises about sex as well as other aspects of their relationships. At this step, problems with give and take can become apparent. There are some partners who are happy to provide what their partner desires, but they either don't know, they can't ask for, or they can't graciously receive what they want in return. There are also those who don't know how to reciprocate, who can't ascertain what their partners need or graciously give it to them. Over and over again in working with couples, I've seen that being purely a giver or purely a taker (even if you and your partner are complementary in this regard) simply doesn't work over time. Sex, like conflict, is two-sided. There is also the problem of not being able to say no to your partner when what they want or need is something you're not willing to do, whether temporarily or permanently. It may seem on the surface like this wouldn't be an issue, but it is. When one partner does things they don't want to do just to please the other, eventually the resentment mounts. It's important to remember that your partner is not forcing you to do what you don't want to do. If you've never expressed reticence about doing something, you're the one forcing yourself to do what you don't want to do in that circumstance. So it's hardly fair to take it out on your partner later.

The next step in work with couples, once they're no longer at each other's jugulars, is to begin to help them learn to do things (or start to do them again) that will rekindle their sexual life together: Dates, flirting, affectionate touching, love letters, seduction, using erotica, trying new things together, and role playing can be effective strategies for rekindling sex initially as well as keeping it on track. Having good sex depends on feeling safe enough to take risks with your partner without the fear of retaliation or rejection. It's the ultimate form of creative play when all goes well. When the stakes are low and the focus is on fun, love and lust rather than performance, there's no real danger of failure. Carol and Ted, much improved as they came to the end of a six-month-long couples treatment with me, decided to try having sex in the back seat of the car like they had in high school. Though they concluded in the end that the risk of discovery made them anxious rather than excited and learned that they were somewhat more arthritic than they were in their younger days, they ended up laughing and acting silly together. They had a great time together, even though the experience wasn't the stuff of their torrid romantic youth. Mutual sexual expression is the highest form of communication between people, and it has the capacity to take things within a relationship in all sorts of unexpected and interesting directions.

The final step in couples therapy involves having an eye toward the prevention of future problems. By the time you've made the journey through this process, you've already learned the skills you need to avoid future problems. But a therapist can also help you formalize your preventive efforts. Weekly dates as well as meetings to explore how things are going can be helpful. Making sure that the relationship, including sex, remains a priority after treatment can involve re-adjusting your lifestyle and your priorities to make sure. This can involve planning regular meetings to discuss how things are going, as well as regular dates to have sex and to enjoy each other's company. It can involve generating key words that you use as code when you believe that your conversations are veering off into dangerous or unfruitful directions and code words that are shared, private expressions between you. One couple I treated started to say "Let's head north again" whenever they thought they were beginning to hit below the belt in discussions and "Wanna fly south?" when they were feeling in the mood for sex. Variations on the theme evolved over time, so that "going to Mexico" meant oral sex and "going to Texas" meant Carol on top, a kind of riding of the bull, rodeo-style event. Silly? Sure. Fun? Definitely. Sexy? Maybe not to you, but when these code words carry strong emotional connotations and pack the punch of enjoyable past experience, they can be electrifying to those involved.

COUPLES AND VIAGRA

Viagra will change the landscape for many couples. Sexual problems between two people are complicated, because they involve a delicate balance of psychological factors, the interplay of two people's minds. The psychological problems that produce erectile dysfunction can come up rapidly, like storm squalls, or they can be simmering problems that evolve over time. They can be the result of conflicted fantasies and feelings within one individual or arise from problems between partners or some combination of both. Whatever their cause, once erectile problems are established, they can definitely begin to create secondary problems with communication in even the closest and most stable of couples. Viagra can change all that, but what will it do to the delicate balance between the psyches and fantasies of men and women in the bedroom?

Sex between couples is about much more than sex. As Robert Kolodny, medical director of the Behavior Medicine Institute in New Canaan and author of *Heterosexuality* says, "The conjugal bed is often not just an amorous place but a place where anger and resentment get played out in various ways. Sex is not just about physical interaction, but about emotional dynamics too. So while Viagra may give better erections, it does little to address the underlying intimacy issues, communication problems, power struggles, issues of trust."

Others, such as Eileen Palace, director of the Sexual Health Clinic at Tulane University, see Viagra as a way for people to short-circuit the psychological problems that can cause erectile dysfunction. As she puts it, "People today expect things to happen on demand. You can't make sex happen on demand; it's not a fax. Penises are actually very good barometers. They are indicators of what is happening in a relationship."

In discussing the problem, Forrest Sawyer, hosting Nightline, questioned whether Viagra would actually provide a kind of security blanket for men who can't distinguish between sexual performance and actual intimacy, as if a pumped up penis must signal a great relationship. It's for reasons like these that Eileen Palace says Viagra should not be used without therapy: "It's much more likely to be effective when you combine the psychological and medical treatments." If she's right, that would closely parallel our experiences with Prozac and psychotherapy, where combined treatment confers more benefit than either treatment alone.

Viagra may show us, ironically, that some men and women don't want the return of sexual functioning at all. You may have noticed that I've been acting throughout this chapter as if all men and women want the resumption of erections and intercourse. But when one wife of a male patient realized that he would probably become more assertive and interested in sex, she recoiled and said, "But he's too interested already." Viagra may produce that reaction in many couples.

Some therapists are even afraid that Viagra will be detrimental to couples. Pioneering sex therapist David Schnarch, author of *Passionate Marriage,* believes that "better sexual functioning can actually destabilize a relationship." He anticipates Viagra bringing to the surface all sorts of "underlying issues that the couple is not prepared to deal with, such as the case where a man suddenly makes unwanted demands on his wife, or couples in which a woman's weight gain has helped her hide from the question of whether she wants to stay with him and given her a way to blame herself for potency problems." Many therapists even anticipate that males with instant, new-found sexual prowess may want to stray from a dysfunctional marriage, pack up and take their Viagra with them. Dr. Diane Brashear, sex and marriage therapist at Indiana University, believes that "where the real revolution is going to happen [is] that as men can get more aroused very easily, then, in a sense, this puts women on notice to be more sexually responsive. And many women who are married to the men who have had erectile dysfunction . . . are used to having a partner who is not interested in sex or who is not able to perform. And so what this is going to do is really change the balance of a relationship."

Chief NBC medical correspondent Dr. Bob Arnot believes Viagra will create a huge disparity in which "millions and millions of men in their late forties and fifties and sixties will have the sexual performance of a twenty-five- or thirty-year-old. And if there isn't a drug for their mates, and their mates feel that they aren't able to catch up, think of the social ramifications, in terms of marriages that don't make it, in terms of men who then will have more of a roving eye than they've had anytime since they were twenty or twenty-five years of age. So with any sort of major breakthrough like this, there's apt to be major social upheaval, and I think we're only beginning to see what some of the negative outcomes of this could be."

It's simply too soon to tell how Viagra may affect different couples' sexual lives together. But changing the balance of a relationship does not necessarily mean changing it for the worse. Sure, Viagra may shake up a couple's usual dynamics—it may even precipitate a crisis. But as the Chinese saying goes, "in crisis, opportunity." From my perspective, what will really tell how Viagra affects a couple will depend upon how they've handled the period of impotence as well as what they're prepared to do to get their sexual relationship back on track.

If Viagra seems to derail things further or points up new areas of conflict in your relationship, there's a good chance that therapy can help. Becoming less depressed with Prozac had unexpected and sometimes adverse consequences for people long involved in relationships that had been built around or had adapted to their depression and dependence.

That doesn't necessarily mean those relationships can't re-equilibrate given a chance and a helping hand.

Viagra may be the miracle drug that guarantees an erection for a man, but psychotherapy may be needed to get him and his partner back to dancing close together cheek to cheek.

PART III

Women and Viagra

9

Women Speak Out About
Men and Viagra

While men across America have been romping to their druggists like frolicking puppies slobbering over a new bone, some women seem to have been spending their time being catty. Admittedly, the men's sound bites have lacked originality: They've been short, affirmative, and boring, the kind of quotes men give when they're eager to get back to playing with that new bone. Women have been more verbose. It seems as if women have taken the emergence of erectile dysfunction and Viagra as an opportunity to comment on how they really feel about men, penises, and sex. The women writing headlines across the country have been uniformly catty, but it seems that the wives of men with erectile dysfunction are taking a wait-and-see attitude. This chapter will look at the themes about men, women and sex that have been steadily emerging since Viagra's release and the reality behind the humor.

"I have some trepidation about it," Diane admitted readily. "You can't quite tell how the drug's going to shake things up. I also have faith in Bernie. He is the man I married and I've loved him all these years. With everyone talking about the effects of Viagra on men, though, I get worried."

It's not surprising Diane would feel apprehensive, since if we're to believe the media perspective, Viagra has simply highlighted certain fundamental truths about men: They're phallocentric and ruled by their penises. As *New York Times* columnist Maureen Dowd put it, "Men think women are greeting the arrival of Viagra, which promises to enhance performance if taken an hour before sex, with as much unalloyed glee as they are. Sorry, guys, but it's more complicated than that. Women already think men are led too much by their anatomy."

Diane White, writing in the *Boston Globe*, assumed the role of Miss Manners to address the inevitable social sticky points that'll come up with Viagra. The question: "I am about to take Viagra for the first time. My partner is aware of this. Is there any sort of etiquette involved?" The answer: "Try to include her in the experience. Allow her to think that she played some role, however small, in your arousal. Don't say at the outset, 'This is an experiment.' Don't try to see how many times you can do it in an hour. Don't say 'Hurry up, I want to get my money's worth.' When you're finished don't jump up and down on the bed shouting, 'Whoopee!' If at the end she applauds, accept it with as much grace and humility as you can muster."

White as much as says that men are sexually inept and don't know the first thing about women and pleasure. Merrill Markoe, writer and humorist, author of *A Guide to Love,* concurs: "Did you ever notice the fact that men who can take a car apart and put it back together have no idea where anything is on a woman? You need some kind of a manual to give to men that goes with the Viagra." Those writers are paid to make jokes, but other columnists seem to be agreeing more earnestly that men just don't know much about sex and pleasing women. Dr. Ruth notes that "Even if a man has an erection from floor to ceiling and can keep it that way for an hour, it will not be pleasurable for a woman if he is not sexually literate." Another sex therapist said that American men "see being sexual as having intercourse. We're a very meat and potatoes culture. In other cultures they toss in a few mushrooms."

Other columnists seem to have used Viagra as an opportunity to advance the idea that women know what's really wrong with men—and it's not impotence, and what men really need—and it's not Viagra. Ellen Goodman, writing in *The Baltimore Sun* says, "I can't help wondering why we got a pill to help men with performance instead of communication." Maureen Dowd had another suggestion for all those downtrodden firms that Pfizer has left in the dust, a kind of women's fantasia on pharmaceuticals of the future. "We are still dreaming of pills that would increase male self-awareness instead of self-indulgence. An unscientific poll of my girlfriends found that they would rather have a pill that could change a man's personality an hour after sex. A pill that insures that he always calls the next day and never gets spooked."

"If Pfizer's rivals are smart," Dowd continues, "they're looking for the Viagra antidote. For each woman who celebrates Viagra, there's another who has nightmares about her sixty-two-year old husband undergoing a satyric transformation and chasing twenty-one-year-old interns, his desk littered with empty Viagra bottles. Few wives want to worry about counting their husbands' Viagra pills. And think of the male wrath if women get out of the mood during that crucial window of Viagra opportunity."

The columnists that write about women's issues are chiming in predictably. Maureen Downey, a writer for the *Atlanta Journal,* asks: "Hasn't our national 'Sex Lies and Audiotape' scandal shown us that men (aside from those with genuine medical problems) need a cold shower more than a thrill pill? If men want to firm up something, they could start with that secondary organ known as the brain.

"If guys are gulping the pills to impress women, I have news: Men don't have to swing from the bedpost to prove they're Tarzan. They can just hoist a few garbage bags out to the curb."

Then there's the perspective that Viagra is just the

kind of thing that men would dream up and Wall Street would love. Erica Jong called Viagra "the perfect American medicament. It raises the Dow Jones and the penis, too. If you were ever wondering whether the stock market was a metaphor for male potency, here's your answer." Ellen Goodman, among others, seemed to see Viagra's development as a kind of male conspiracy: "How is it possible that we came up with a male impotence pill before we got a male birth-control pill? The Vatican, you will note, has approved Viagra while still condemning condoms."

"It also seems," Goodman continued, "that in some places we'll get health insurance coverage for male potency before we get female contraceptives. Hasn't anyone noticed that the chief sexual turnoff for women is fear of pregnancy? It's enough to give a girl Viagra envy."

The tone of all these statements, simply put, is that the battle between the sexes continues. Women and men are still fighting like cats and dogs. And Pfizer, for its part, understands the power that women have. It has said that when the time comes, it will advertise the drug in women's magazines. Those savvy Pfizer execs know that even if it's men who have the penile problem, it's often women who wear the pants about these things. Men play the game, as the old saying goes, but women know the score. The emergent message from all this media meowing is that women, of course, are clearly the superior and dominant sex. Consider Camille Paglia's perspective: "The erection is the last gasp of modern manhood. If men can't continue to produce erections, they're going to evolve themselves right out of the human species. I want men to really examine why they need this pill. It's like the steel they would get if they were at war." Once men's erections were like steel. Now it's the Viagra that is.

Nancy Friday feels that it must be frightening to be a male these days: "We're a performance-oriented society, and sex has always been to the women's advantage." Erica Jong's 1973 *Fear of Flying* committed by her account "the ultimate literary faux pas" of revealing that even tough guys were not always hard. Now, she believes, the more sexually demanding and harder women got, the softer the men became. "But erections were starting to get iffy as women were starting to demand sexual pleasure," Jong writes. "The game had begun to change. Men were expected to please women as women had once been expected to please men. This made a lot of men very nervous—nervous enough to lose their erections." Even Bob Guccione, publisher of *Penthouse,* agrees: "I think to a great extent men have felt emasculated as a result of the original feminist agenda." Both Jong and Guccione seem to think that Viagra can begin to even the score. Jong feels Viagra is the great antidote to female superiority, to that fabulous "all-weather cunt" that is "always there, always ready. The same cunt that, to feminists, is what leads men to invent the myth of female inadequacy in the first place." Guccione concurs, stating that Viagra will free the American male libido from the emasculating doings of feminists. Erica Jong and Bob Guccione in bed together? Maybe Viagra *is* the solution to the war between the sexes.

As Freud knew early on, humor is a defense, a way of both expressing and protecting oneself from an unpleasant fantasy. So what are the fantasies behind the catty humor that women have engaged in about Viagra? I asked this question of women on an Internet site and got some pretty consistent answers, some recurring themes. I've selected several to show you what women really think about Viagra. What are they really worried about?

Phallocentricity and a sense of being left out, becoming auxiliary, or otherwise unimportant topped the list of fears commonly cited by women. Like Barbara, a forty-six-year-old who wrote: "Of course I'm glad he's happy but I also see a big problem looming. (We've yet to talk about it. Maybe this is all just a start-up reaction and will go away in time.) The problem in a nutshell is this: Making love now feels like Jack's having an affair with his penis. Here's he and his dick, balling it up, pleased as punch with themselves. I feel like I've been left out of it altogether. Jack's problem wasn't so severe to begin with. I mean, I know he was bothered about being less hard and all, but I felt we'd adapted very well. Perhaps it was just our greater emotional maturity after twenty-four years of marriage, or the fact that the kids were out of the house. But making love in the last few years had become, in certain ways, more satisfying for us; well, that's what I thought. Jack had grown more playful, being in bed wasn't some stud-fest, but funny and fun. One of the things that we had started doing a lot, on his initiation, I might add, was cunnilingus, and that was very, very nice.

"Since Viagra," Barbara continued, "it's just intercourse, intercourse straight up, and to me it all feels like a marathon. Jack got it up three times last night but I felt for all the world like he was monitoring his progress with a stopwatch and a ruler. It was like there was a whole squad of cheerleaders in his head, the ones who drove me nuts when we were in high school. Meanwhile I felt like chopped liver. I've seen on the Internet women talking about their concerns. Is it the drug, they wonder, or is it me? I think the answer to that is clear, at least in my household: It's the drug, at least for the moment. I could be an inflatable doll and Jack wouldn't care. In fact he might prefer it if she were slim-hipped like I used to be. So I bide my time and hope that Jack will get off of his cloud.

"Meanwhile, I've concluded that Viagra is a drug by men and for men. The only advantage I can see is having him keep that erection longer for me. I read somewhere that men climax in about two minutes whereas women take six or more. So I guess it could be good in the end if I can get it through Jack's thick skull that my ideal Romeo isn't Leonardo DiCaprio at eighteen. It's him the way he used to be, last month before Viagra."

Related to the return of men's interest in sex were the concerns of some women that their mates would find them less attractive as sexual partners, or would want to be with women who never knew that they'd had a problem in the first place. Many women felt the effects of turning back their husband's clocks on their own assessments of how they had aged, not to mention how their husband's impotence had affected their lives and their waistlines. As they confronted saddle bags and crow's feet, some seemed to have a sinking feeling that if their husbands were really eighteen again, they'd be headed to Weight Watchers at least, if not divorce court. It was as if the ball had been thrown back into their court, by husbands who'd had to struggle with issues of self-esteem, attractiveness and vulnerability in the wake of their erectile dysfunction. Now they were the ones facing the issues themselves. The tables had been turned, sexually speaking. Related to these concerns were worries about infidelity, abandonment, even HIV. I also noted in some responses a sense of angry entitlement. These women had stayed with men that they secretly viewed as damaged goods for many years. Now that their husband's erectile dysfunction was better, they'd better be loyal. Secretly, I suspected, they wondered if they could really keep up with the sexual demands of their new and improved partners—and whether they wanted to.

Lisa wrote from her home in Nebraska to tell me about her experiences with the drug. "I'm a sixty-eight-year-old retired high school English teacher who has lived with my husband Frank for almost fifty years. When we were in our teenage days and our twenties, we sometimes had sex five times a week. But over the years with kids, a mortgage, both of our jobs and our church duties, our sex life slowly dwindled. I thought that was OK with both of us. We were affectionate with each other, always kissing goodnight. And I thought it was normal for us to start having sex once a week, usually on Friday or Saturday. I never felt it made the earth shake or anything, but I liked the closeness and I could see it was important to Frank. It's still enjoyable even though Frank's sugar problem has affected him in bed. But basically, I feel satisfied with myself and Frank. With our marriage and how it's changed over time. We have a lovely family and grandkids underfoot. We're really partners in the way I hoped we'd be when we got married.

"So along comes this pill and it's scary. Frank and I haven't discussed it, but he keeps telling dumb Viagra jokes, the kind of off-color ones that I shush him from saying around the kids. I'm afraid he's going to want to try it. I was happy to let sleeping dogs lie, as they say, but he may insist. I guess I have the feeling that the medicine is going to give me lots of trouble I didn't bargain for. And if he's feeling so much younger, if he changes, maybe his expectations of me will change and I won't be good enough for him anymore.

"I've never worried about it before, but maybe I'll have to now. Maybe he'll want someone younger who can keep up with him sexually. I hope not. He's always been a loving, reasonable man. I'm keeping my fingers crossed. I wish that pill had never been invented because I like things the way they are."

I got one long response from a woman who was actually happy with Viagra. Tired of coping with her husband's impotence, she'd been thinking of having an affair herself, even though she knew she'd feel guilty if she did. But she was deeply frustrated. Now she wondered if the drug could actually save her sex life and maybe her marriage as well.

Using just her E-mail name of JC, she wrote: "I'm happy, happy, happy! And not only do I have this new-found joy in my life but what's striking is how this gift (that's really how I think of it, a gift from on high!) of happy sex reverberates throughout my life in so many seemingly unrelated ways.

"To take a step back it was merely two months ago when I was feeling deeply sad, existential angst, etc., and all that which accompanies being sexually frustrated in an otherwise loving relationship. I think my frustration had grown more profound when I hit forty this year. I had this nagging feeling of, Hey, this is my sexual prime and I'm stuck in a life without passion and I'm going to wake up at sixty-five and . . . The quandary for me in what now seems like a lifetime ago (in March!) was that I truly love my husband, can't imagine a better partner, but my sexual yearnings had become overwhelming and our culture (at least the movies I see) do hold up that 'follow-your-passion' ideal. Like *The Bridges of Madison County*. I can see why Meryl Streep went for that photographer and can feel how bad she must have felt when he left.

"If it weren't for Viagra I don't think I could have stayed faithful. I was bound to stray and then be faced with a painful dilemma. But who ever said fairy tales can't come true! Today sex is outstanding—that's right, from zero to a hundred in no time—outstanding. My husband and I feel like kids in a candy store, gobbling up every sexual escapade we can. In my years of frustration I don't think I dared to realize just how valuable sex is to life, to marriage, to my sense of self, to aging with grace—together. You can bet we're going to cherish and nurture our precious sex for many years to come. If this all sounds like a religious convert, so be it. Hallelujah! Amen."

The women whose lives were radically changed by their husbands' new best friend had been sustained for years on the potency of memories alone. Now they were eager to make new ones. When the hoopla about men and Viagra has died down, women will probably be satisfied with what it's done for their sex lives as they've aged.

Viagra came out just in time for pre–Baby Boomers like Bob Dole and his wife, Elizabeth. Bob is a prostate cancer survivor who admitted he'd been in the clinical trials and said that Viagra had worked well for him. For days no one asked his wife to corroborate. Finally someone asked Elizabeth, in New York for World Red Cross Day. According to *New York Newsday* she "giggled" and said: "Let me just say this. He was in the protocol. And it's a great drug." So far no one has gotten up the nerve to ask her if she's tried it herself. Her answer, I imagine, will be a seasoned "No comment." For many of the women with husbands for whom Viagra has worked, there is no need to be catty. They're too busy purring instead. And some of them are contemplating taking the drug themselves. The next chapter will look at the women who are pioneering the use of Viagra in women, especially in postmenopausal women.

10

Women Taking Viagra

Women are not necessarily fair when it comes to men, their penises, and Viagra. Perhaps they're just jealous. But they won't have to be for long. The biggest story since men and Viagra is women and Viagra—and what the drug can offer women is likely to be even bigger than what it has given men.

For one thing, there are the numbers: A recent study reported in *Newsweek* suggested that more than one-third of women 18 to 59 experience sexual dysfunction, compared with just 10% of men. Women also have sexual difficulties earlier in life in higher numbers. Just as with aging men, arteriosclerosis and diabetes in aging women impair blood flow leading to vaginal dryness, which in turn causes pain during intercourse along with the lack of clitoral engorgement that accompanies arousal. The advent of menopause also decreases vaginal lubrication and causes gradual thinning of the delicate tissues of the vulva, the outer areas of the female genitalia that surround the vaginal opening, as well as thinning and increased fragility of the walls of the vagina itself. These changes can make intercourse painful and cause women to use artificial vaginal lubricants to try to compensate for the changes wrought by estrogen depletion. Throughout the life cycle, intercourse is stacked against women's orgasms, with men on average taking about 20% of the time women do to reach orgasm. While Viagra won't by any means guarantee orgasm, it may help. As NBC medical correspondent Bob Arnot recently argued, women have a greater pelvic blood flow requirement for sex than men do, so, theoretically, Viagra could have an even more important effect on women than it does on men.

I wanted to hear how Viagra affected women other than my patient Jane, but since it is not yet approved for use in women, I would not yet suggest it even to females that I thought might benefit. I wanted to gather stories about what its effects in women felt like firsthand.

Interestingly, there was no shortage of female friends who had decided to try the drug, getting it from boyfriends and spouses. My friend Lisa was head of the pack, as usual. She reported at first that Viagra gave her a whopping headache that made it hard to concentrate on whether sex was better or not. But on her second run, when she took Viagra with ibuprofen, her response was much better. "It felt like my clitoris would burst," she reported. "And my vagina was definitely boggy. I couldn't decide if I liked it or I didn't, but it was definitely much wetter. I guess it taught me there's such a thing as being too lubricated. But I can imagine it working well for women who have a real problem." For Lisa the real difference was that she felt her clitoris was much more sensitive, that a mere suggestion of a touch produced a little volley of orgasms. "I don't know for sure if they're worth $10 or not. My orgasms were good before, just different. Still, I think you could safely say Viagra 'worked' for me."

Considering embryonic anatomy, it's actually not surprising that if Viagra works for men it might help women. After all, we all start out the same in terms of what types of tissues we have, even if the shapes and forms they take differ between genders. Males and females are actually identical at week six of fetal development, when both have a genital tubercle which elongates greatly in men to produce the phallus and elongates to a lesser extent in women to produce the clitoris. The clitoris contains tissue that is embryonically the same in origin as the penis, composed of the equivalent of the corpus cavernosum and the corpus spongiosum. In fact, the glans clitoris or "hood" of the clitoris is the embryonic equivalent of the glans penis or "head" of the penis. Another embryonic structure, the urethral folds, fuse in males to form the penile urethra while the folds remain unfused in women, forming the labia minora or inner lips, which in turn make up the vestibule, or opening to the vagina. Meanwhile, the so-called genital swellings form the scrotum in men and the labia majora, or outer lips, in women.

In other ways, male and female genital development is quite different. At a certain point in development, both men and women have both Wolffian and Muellerian ducts. The Wolffian ducts, under the influence of testosterone in would-be boys, form the testes, prostate gland, epididymis, vas deferens and seminal vesicles. The Wolffian duct gives rise to the ovaries, but in the absence of testosterone, it degenerates, even in women who will later run with the wolves. The Muellerian ducts, which degenerate in men, take over in women to form the vagina, cervix, uterus, and fallopian tubes. This entire process is completed by around eight weeks of fetal development.

Despite these inner, developmental differences, the stages of the sexual response cycle in men and women are thought to be the same. You may recall that establishing these similarities despite the obvious anatomical differences was one of Masters and Johnson's big contributions. In both sexes, desire—the wish to engage in sexual behavior—is followed by arousal. In both sexes, arousal means increased heart rate, increased blood pressure, skin flushing due to vasodilation, and the overall increase in blood flow to the genitals known as vasocongestion. In men, this increased blood flow results in erections. In women it does, too—clitoral erections, that is. The clitoris is the female organ that's analogous to the penis in men, erectile tissue, nerve endings and all. The clitoris also happens to be the only organ on any part of the bodies of men and women that is apparently there simply for pleasure. The urethra, which carries both urine and semen, runs through the penis, making its job like that of a fireman with a hose. Meanwhile the clitoris just sits there, waiting to be amused.

Viagra just may tickle its fancy.

It did for Katie, anyway. "It's the best thing since Ecstasy!" she proclaimed. "What drugs like Ecstasy do for desire, Viagra does for getting wet and being able to come. I felt like I could come for hours, and it's usually hard for me. But I felt embarrassed to tell my boyfriend that I had taken it, because he was so into thinking that all those orgasms were him. They were him and they weren't. They were him on Viagra."

The second aspect of arousal in women is vaginal wall swelling, which is the result of increased blood flow to the pelvic area more generally. Then there's secretion of fluids from two sets of glands called the cervical and vestibular glands. The equivalent of this stage in men is emission, or movement, of the sperm from the testes and epididymis to the vas deferens, where they get set to be ejaculated during orgasm. So Viagra might promote vaginal lubrication at the same time as it engorges the clitoris and vagina with blood, making the sensations in both exquisitely sensitive. In theory, that's what Viagra can do during the arousal stage of the sexual response cycle in women.

Orgasm, the third stage of sexual response, is also a parallel stage of sexual response in men and women with two notable exceptions: First, orgasms—the rhythmic contractions of pelvic muscles—are punctuated by ejaculation in men. Second, men have a longer refractory period between orgasms. Women are capable of being multiorgasmic within a short period of time. The jury is still out on whether the increased arousal that Viagra produces puts men and women closer to orgasm as well. The official party line of Pfizer is that Viagra neither increases desire, the first stage, nor does it affect orgasm, the third stage. It works solely by increasing arousal, the second stage.

It may turn out, though, that Viagra redefines the stages of the sexual response cycle.

"Many women struggle with the desire issue," says Dr. Diane Brashear, a sex and marriage therapist at Indiana University, "and they're looking for some kind of magical pill that makes them turn on a lot easier." In other words, they have problems with the first stage, desire. So, what if Viagra helps with more than just the arousal phase? "I think the whole Viagra situation is going to raise a lot of questions for us who do counseling," Brashear continues, "because we've always assumed that one has to have sexual interest or appetite first before you get arousal. The question now is, if you can take a pill to get arousal, is it going to then make you more interested in having sex?"

If Viagra increases arousal, will it also make it

easier for men and women to climax? As a psychiatrist, I think that there's a problem with separating out desire as a discrete step of the response cycle anyway, since if you interfere with desire at any stage of the sexual response cycle (except, perhaps, the moment before orgasm) you can shut it down. That's why women who urinate or defecate while being raped sometimes make the rapist stop: the sexual response is not so automatic that something designed to grossly interfere with desire doesn't have an impact. As I've tried to convey throughout this book, mind matters across the entire cycle.

Jennie's experiences with Viagra suggested that it was the permission to be sexually wild more than a specific effect such as increased lubrication or more clitoral engorgement that made Viagra work for her. "I think when I took it I was expecting something big to happen. And I guess I felt like I could be a little more wild with my husband Max. It was like a kind of passport to being a slutty girl that I seemed to really get off on. I couldn't really tell you if it was more than that." Jennie's story reminded me that women, perhaps even more than men, have to struggle to feel sexually free.

Despite the cautions of researchers that Viagra would not help with problems of desire, within two weeks of Viagra's release for men, the rush to use it and test it in women (in that order) was on. It was clear that plenty of women had enough desire—for the pill, at least—to go to great lengths to get it. One enthralled female Internet user who created a special site devoted to Viagra for women bills the drug as: "The perfect and most thoughtful gift for your girlfriend." She expounds upon the urgent need for approval for women, meanwhile giving us a home-made anatomy lesson of sorts. Men, it turns out, are just women turned inside out. "The male scrotum is the same as the female vagina, only turned inside out . . . The female clitoris has the same number of nerve endings as the penis, only they're packed into a smaller space." Her description is inaccurate since it's the scrotum and the labia majora or outer lips that are analogous. Then comes her call to arms, as she tells all husbands and boyfriends to "go down to the doctor and tell him that *you* are having difficulties and . . . then give it to your girlfriend!"

Sexpert Susie Bright was soon in on the action as well, providing all the stats from the first female celebrity test drive of Viagra. Sex differences were evident as early as the headlines. "Viagra calls: My date with the wonder drug" she entitled her spin. One date and already Susie had decided that Viagra was the type who calls. Sure her vagina was extra puffy, but that doesn't mean Viagra wasn't a gentleman. "I could have another orgasm," she writes, "I'm sure I could, but I'm on deadline now, and after all, I swallowed this pill for research, for science, not just to take another busman's holiday. My pussy may still be puffy, but I have a greater goal in mind."

Bright's other comments may actually be more

telling. She reports, for instance, that now, after having children, she often finds herself turning away from some compelling turn-on when she feels the tug of non-erotic obligations. In fact, she spent the night before the test drive up all night with her second-grade daughter, who was throwing up. Not the type of thing that would inspire most women to really let loose in bed. And having time alone with her lover on a weekday morning was obviously at least part of the turn-on of Viagra for her. But there were also real physical differences, starting with the fact that her vulva was more royal purple than pink in color. Then she noticed that nipple stimulation was more arousing, that she can orgasm while performing 69, and that she had multiple orgasms. But Bright doesn't seem to see the production of arousal as producing anything like guaranteed sexual desire. She agrees with Pfizer that it's not an aphrodisiac: "If you're an uptight bitch, you're still going to be an uptight bitch an hour after taking it, albeit with a LOT of extra vasocongestion." The only unexpected side effect she experienced was that her chronic low back pain was gone. Increased vasocongestion, perhaps?

Viagra's use in women was tested by more than just your sporadic Internet sex star as well. After initially disavowing interest in the pill for women, Pfizer finally admitted that, yes, it too had thought of Viagra for women and was conducting clinical trials. I suppose it's good if you're the king of pharmaceuticals not to look like you're out to take over the entire world in one fell swoop. Better to start with half and wait a few days before making it clear that you're after the women, too.

European trials are reportedly under way by Pfizer, with five hundred postmenopausal British women who have problems with vaginal lubrication involved in its Phase II trials being conducted at Pfizer's UK headquarters in Sandwich, Kent. U.S. trials are also supposedly planned. Pfizer's being very hush-hush about the data from their clinical trials in Britain, saying only that the data has not yet been analyzed.

Even if the data show that Viagra helps women, Pfizer will have to reapply for FDA approval for use in women. Why is Pfizer being so quiet, giving no timetable at all for the possibility of Viagra for women? Probably because of the thorny medico-legal problems they face in attempting to study the drug's effects on fertility, pregnancy, and offspring of women who took it. All those -genicities we talked about in Chapter 6 come into play. To get approval for use in women, Pfizer will have to study much more than Chinese hamsters—they'll need human female guinea pigs, including pregnant ones.

Viagra has non-Pfizer physicians interested as well. In mid-April about one hundred urologists, gynecologists, sex therapists, and drug representatives met to discuss female impotence. Talk about male impotence coming out of the closet with this drug, female impotence was practically unheard of until now.

Some of these physicians are already conducting studies on Viagra for female impotence. At Robert Wood Johnson Medical School in New Jersey, researchers have given it to women to measure their physiological responses while watching pornographic movies. At Loyola University in Maywood, Illinois, sexual dysfunction researchers have set up a protocol to test the drug among women. "We have just started exploring women and Viagra," says Dr. John Mulhall, a researcher and director of the Male Sexual Health Clinic. Already one in three calls have been from women interested in whether the drug can help them. But, he notes, most of the women are not candidates because most female dysfunction is related to orgasm or libido. "Viagra doesn't address those issues," he notes. Dr. Margaret Wierman, chief of endocrinology and assistant professor of medicine at the University of Colorado Health Sciences Center, concurs. She warns: "It's very scary for physicians to be hammered by patients for drugs we haven't seen studies on."

As for females and Viagra, she notes, "We don't know what controls the libido." Viagra may increase blood flow to the female sex organs, "but no one knows what role clitoral erection plays in a woman's sexual response."

Not all doctors feel the need to be so circumspect. Dr. Irwin Goldstein, a renowned Boston University School of Medicine urologist, made it clear that he isn't waiting until the data are all in to use Viagra in women whom he feels could benefit. He admits already prescribing Viagra to women, an off-label (non-FDA approved) drug. His colleague, Jennifer Berman, a urology expert at the University of Maryland School of Medicine, believes that there are as many "impotent women"—women who don't enjoy sex because of poor lubrication or other physiological factors—as men. "It makes sense it would work in women too. Blood flow equates with sexual arousal in them too."

Berman currently has ten women on Viagra in an unofficial pilot study. She is not funded in any way by Pfizer, so her patients self-pay—gladly, she notes. She's getting many calls every day from women who so badly want help from her. In a bold and unusual move, all of the women in her study are young and pre-menopausal. They have all had hysterectomies and most had some form of sexual dysfunction related to the surgery afterward. This makes them safer research subjects, since they won't inadvertently get pregnant while participating in the trial. Since the potential risks to a human fetus from Viagra have not been established, researchers usually stick to post-menopausal women if possible.

Berman reports that all of her women, on 50 or 100 mg, have had excellent results—all of them. Some women who were completely anorgasmic—unable to reach orgasm even through masturbation—have now been able to have an orgasm for the first time. And while not every single female has attained this result, the women universally report heightened sensation, saying things like "it feels much more sensitive all over down there." All have clitoral engorgement and vaginal lubrication responses to Viagra, making it as much the Pfizer flow pill as the Pfizer riser.

Berman notes that she doesn't know exactly how and why Viagra effects orgasm. "I have insight into how Viagra works in erections in men, and how it works to increase blood flow, engorgement and lubrication in women, but the scientific community doesn't really have a basis for understanding the circuitry and mechanics of the female orgasm." Viagra, she notes, may help us learn more.

Berman has also received an $88,000 grant from the American Foundation for Urological Diseases for scientific research on Viagra, to examine its molecular biology, to conduct tissue analyses, and to do animal studies. (Animal studies? How do you measure the turn-on factor in rats?) Berman stimulates female rabbits and rats electrically while they're sleeping, then measures changes in blood flow, vaginal wall pressure and vaginal lubrication. These may just be the only creatures on the planet that sleep through their first Viagra test drives. Berman also creates animal models designed to mimic the conditions that might affect sexual arousal in women, such as clamping the aorta in a rat to mimic effects of atherosclerosis. Then she does extensive vaginal cell cultures, measures nitric oxide, and generally tries to ascertain the effects of an interruption of blood flow on the various parts of the female genital system. It's because of these scientific studies on animals and the positive results of her early trials on women that she feels so confident that Viagra will help women, too.

In July, Berman and her mentor Goldstein will begin testing Viagra in post-menopausal women, a group who often have problems with lubrication. One of the women is so desperate that she is paying thousands of dollars to travel from California to Maryland to take part in the tests. In true corporate form, Pfizer has exempted itself from any responsibility for the use of Viagra in women, and both doctors are therefore assuming a big risk in prescribing it to women. But Berman feels so certain of its efficacy based on animal and human male trials and preliminary data in women. The clitoris, she reiterates, "is exactly the same tissue as the penis." As a female urologist, Berman feels a sense of "personal responsibility" to do this work: "It's a very male-dominated field and I really feel it's my role, my responsibility, to do this for women. I really want to help women.

"People just don't appreciate that women's sexual functioning affects relationships the way that a man's does." Berman notes that one of her female patients in her twenties was so different following a hysterectomy, so disinterested in sex, that her husband was convinced she was having an affair. Her patient had great results with Viagra, putting the question of infidelity in this case to rest. Then there was the woman who was just so tired of faking it with her boyfriend that she decided to come clean.

For her, Berman reports, "Viagra was a vindication. Everyone had just been advising her to 'take a warm bath, relax' and that advice was just frustrating her more and more." But now she's happy because of how well Viagra works.

It seems likely that Viagra will not be the only "impotence" drug that will become available to women in the near future. Vasomax, the oral form of phentolamine being tested by Zonagen, may also help by increasing pelvic blood flow. In addition, Spontane (Apomorphine), which works on the central nervous system rather than on smooth muscle constriction, will soon be available. Male trials of both drugs are near completion and trials in women are planned. Likewise, prostaglandin creams such as Topiglan, which are applied to the skin surface of the penis or vulva to stimulate blood flow, may also work in women, and trials in women are supposed to start after those in men are finished. Women are indeed the second sex as far as pharmaceutical companies are concerned: men's trials first and then women's. It's no wonder that so many women have been catty about Viagra for men. But the new impotence drugs for women are in the pipeline, and while many women may not want to wait, Dr. Berman encourages them to try. "We need female subjects who've never taken the drug before to try it on," she notes. There is also the thorny issue of whether Viagra adversely affects fertility or the course of pregnancy or the health of offspring."

There's a political issue as well: Will Pfizer spend

the money and put itself at legal risk to get the drug approved in women, or will it look the other way if women are already being given Viagra by their physicians, leaving the individual physicians open to risk? Without FDA approval for use in women, insurance companies will be hesitant to cover even a part of it, the way they are considering covering Viagra for men. This is a new issue in off-label drug use. For years, psychiatrists prescribed Prozac for patients with panic disorder and obsessive-compulsive disorder even before Eli Lilly got FDA approval for using the drug for these indications. The drug had been approved solely for the treatment of depression. It was impossible for a pharmacist or an insurance company to tell for what reason the drug was actually being prescribed, so they covered it. Now with Viagra, all a pharmacist or insurance company has to do is figure out the sex of the person for whom it is being prescribed and the fact that the use is off-label is immediately obvious. So insurance companies can easily turn down prescriptions from women even if their physicians feel that the drug is being used for a genuine medical condition for which it is the appropriate choice. It's a brave new world of insurance regulations to contend with.

Perhaps the woman I know who was the happiest about Viagra was my friend Kathy. A lesbian in a relationship of eight years, she and her girlfriend Annie had been feeling left out of the Viagra craze in its early days. At first they pretended not to care, to be above it all and not to need the drug. "After all," they said smugly, "our penises are always ready anyway. And they're detachable and come in a wide range of colors, shapes and sizes. Strap them on, take them off. We can keep them in a box by the bed and they don't talk back. Plus, having an erect penis around here doesn't cost $10 a pop." Now, they figured, a straight woman could enjoy what a lesbian had always taken for granted: a partner with an erection that lasted as long as she wanted it to. But I was also not surprised to see them decide to ride the wave after the Viagra for women story broke. For Kathy, Viagra enabled her to reach orgasm from cunnilingus alone, something she'd never been able to do before. Annie was impressed by the degree of vaginal sensitivity she had, since in general she did not like vaginal penetration. Now, with Viagra, it felt better. "If I wasn't so sure about its physical effects on each of us," Kathy quipped, "I'd be convinced that what we both really wanted was to be included in the Viagra craze. It seemed for a while there that lesbians were the only ones who wouldn't benefit. It didn't seem right. And," Annie continued triumphantly, "we don't have to worry about what David Letterman called Viagra's single biggest side effect—pregnancy."

It seems that women straight and gay are getting interested in questions of power and length now as well, the kinds of issues that men have been preoccupied with for years. So maybe sexual prowess and power will take on a new, gender-neutral meaning with Viagra on the scene. If the power to control sexual response is contained in the little mighty pill that is Viagra and pill that works equally well for both men and women, then perhaps the playing field in the war between the sexes will be leveled to a greater extent than ever in history.

It may be that the only thing Viagra can't do for women is give them the ability to pee standing up.

Conclusion: Living and Loving with Viagra

The room buzzed with excited young Pfizer reps, bright-eyed, bushy-tailed salespeople, many of them in their twenties and thirties. They knew they were about to embark on the biggest pharmaceutical launch in history. Then the meeting was called to order and, as the reps watched, actors portrayed the lives of men with impotence and their partners. It was Pfizer's attempt at sensitivity training for reps, an attempt to help its young sales force understand how erectile dysfunction affects men and their partners, what it does to relationships. One middle-aged actor who participated said he believed that after all was said and done, the biggest realization of the afternoon for many of the reps may have been the lesson that people older than they were still having sex. The reps later received tips about handling Viagra jokes at cocktail parties from a brochure that instructed them to "redirect humorous remarks [about Viagra] to more appropriate discussion by not joining in the humor and pointing out the seriousness of the subject matter."

Meanwhile, across the Atlantic, a blue-green haze settled across the lush hills of Ringaskiddy, County Cork, Ireland, a sleepy fishing village poised at the side of the sea. Ringaskiddy's main claim to fame used to be an old stone tower erected by the British to defend against invasion by Napoleon. Now it's better known as one of the main locations where sildenafil—the active ingredient in Viagra—is made. Sildenafil keeps rolling off the production line, bound for bedrooms around the world. Meanwhile the townspeople joke that Ireland is the one place in the world that doesn't need Viagra. Given all that ale, the claim is difficult to believe. Will Viagra make Ringaskiddy a tourist attraction one day, a stop on the guided tour about drugs that changed the world? If so, its old stone tower, never actually needed in the end to fight off Napoleon, may finally take on a useful symbolic meaning.

Within a month of Viagra's release, it was difficult to find someone who hadn't tried it himself or didn't know someone who had. Many erectile exhibitionists—male and female—put their test drives in print, while cartoonists and columnists competed to see who could come up with the most clever lines to capture their audience's over-saturated attentions.

Viagra had already invaded the language, and it

sometimes seemed impossible for the media—from political pundits to sportscasters, weathermen to the fashion police—to get through a sentence without mentioning the new wonder drug:

- "Anyone who says he knows what's going to happen in the NBA playoffs this season has been taking too much Viagra." *(L.A. Times)*
- "Kevin will be our Viagra tablet. He'll get those ratings up," ABC weatherman Spencer Christian said of the new *Good Morning America* host.
- "That was some speech House Speaker Newt Gingrich gave to GOPAC last Monday night in Washington. One might think that somebody had slipped the male potency pill Viagra into his water glass." *(Denver Post)*
- And in the business world, a report in *Barron's* on the boost technology stocks will give to the market reported, "It's a monster dose of Viagra. We're talking virile here."

Another sign that Viagra had immediately been accepted into common parlance, that the Viagratization of America was complete, was the immediate dubbing of the Clinton sex scandal as "Viagra-gate" (despite the common observation that Clinton appeared to be the only man his age in the country who didn't need it). The *Boston Globe* deconstructed the term to its component parts: "Vitality, vigor, virility, virtue—all the v-words from the Latin word 'vir,' which means male." The adverbial, adjectival and verbose possibilities promised to be enough to give William Safire a hard-on for weeks.

Meanwhile the federal government as well as individual states, insurance companies and HMOs scrambled to come up with some reasonable guidelines about how much Viagra would be covered by Medicare, Medicaid and individual insurance plans. They were in effect arguing about how much sex was enough. Florida and Alabama decided on four pills monthly while Louisiana, Arkansas and Maryland cover six. Utah weighed in at ten, perhaps the inevitable legacy of polygamy. But no one could seem to come up with a rationale for their numbers and everyone involved was uneasy and defensive about the prospect that they were regulating sex or sexual satisfaction. Meanwhile, some insurance companies decided that they would pay for the pill only when the prescription was covered by a doctor's note indicating that the erectile dysfunction was real and had been evaluated. And no one seemed to be planning to cover a prescription of the pill made out to a woman.

Behind these wrangles was, of course, money. But some long-time erectile dysfunction sufferers noted that their previous treatments had been even costlier than Viagra. For instance, MUSE costs around $165 for six applications, approximately triple the cost of six Viagra tablets. What would really make the drug expensive would be the increased numbers of patients demanding it, not the absolute cost per prescription.

Viagra raised the Prozac problem in a more dramatic form: Would people without a defined illness, who merely felt better taking the pill than not, indulge in a kind of cosmetic pharmacology? And if they did, should insurance companies pay? The fact that Prozac is a drug for depression, a psychiatric illness, was probably plenty to deter many people, as was the idea that it was monkeying around with brain chemistry. As more and more drugs that improve the quality of life as we age become available, we'll probably face this dilemma again and again. Viagra is a kind of test case for how medicine will be transformed in the next century as it becomes better able to promote health and quality of life rather than just curing illness. Will a sixty-four-year-old who doesn't actually have erectile dysfunction by today's definition but feels better with Viagra on board be viewed as ill or as a substance abuser or user? If Viagra works for him does that mean he has erectile dysfunction after all? Can response to the treatment be considered an indicator of illness? Some have already speculated that Viagra will redefine our understanding of the chemistry of men in midlife, that we will come to appreciate the crucial role of testosterone for men the way we have learned to appreciate estrogen's role in women's health. In fact, the drug may enable us to understand more about sexuality across the life span, allow us to fine-tune our understanding of men's anatomy and physiology as they age. Already evidence is mounting to suggest that testosterone supplements might affect men's bone density and moods. And there's the suggestion that a drug like Viagra can actually prevent the development of erectile dysfunction, a kind of "use-it-or-lose-it" argument.

Of course, the backlash against Viagra was also nearly immediate, with some psychologists warning that Viagra would trigger an increase in impotency as freaked-out men focused on erections grew dependent on the drug. The *L.A. Times* quipped about the need for the formation of a group called WAVE—Workaholics Against Viagra's Effects—which would be a coalition of prominent males from the ranks of corporate CEOs and senior vice presidents, lawyers, investment bankers and admen who saw Viagra as a pernicious threat to the one-hundred-hour workweek.

There were also questions about the role of personal responsibility and whether Viagra would erode it further, with some anticipating that men would invoke the "Viagra" defense as an excuse for affairs or even date rape. Pfizer reportedly worried privately about the possibility of frat parties with a "Viagra" theme, which some college groups quickly made a reality. Then there was the undeniable fact that Viagra could fall into the hands of rapists and pedophiles, people who might use it for evil ends.

Lurking behind many of the issues Viagra has raised is a question about the real nature of men, women and relationships. How will older men want to act if their penises are free to act like they were eighteen again? Will their brains regress, too? Or will they be able to handle their renewed potency with the calm and self-restraint of the sixty-five-year-olds they are? What effect will an eighteen-year-old penis have on a sixty-five-year-old mind? Will there be a rash of divorces, new trophy brides, late-life pregnancies?

As a psychiatrist, I know there are no simple, general answers to these questions. They are the type that can only be answered on a case-by-case basis. People are different in their psyches and souls, in the ways they communicate with their partners and in what their relationships are based upon in the first place. What will determine Viagra's effectiveness and effects will vary widely depending on who's taking it, what they're hoping to achieve and how they and their partner have dealt with the issue of impotence in the first place. As a psychiatrist I also know that the real story is in the details, and I wanted to feel free to probe people's experiences to a greater extent than I felt comfortable doing with my patients. After all, my role in therapy is to help them see what they think. It would be distinctly unusual for me to grill them about their reactions. So I posted inquiries on the worldwide web, hoping to learn more from individuals and their partners who had struggled with impotence. I wanted to be free to speak to them frankly and in detail about their experiences. One group I visited was an on-line support group for prostate cancer survivors and their partners, people who have struggled with a life-threatening illness, all of the treatments for which are known to produce erectile dysfunction.

There I met George and Gigi. Writing from half-way around the world from their humanitarian post in Asia, their story emerged in bits and pieces over the course of our E-mail exchange, with a frankness that would be hard to achieve in a face-to-face interview of strangers. George began the discourse, letting me know that he was sorry some others in his support group were wary of my project and inviting me to begin a "conversation" about "impotence and people and love." I thought that was a promising way to phrase the invitation. He suggested I visit his urologist's web page and take a look at him and his fiancée in the photo gallery so I'd know to whom I was talking. He sent me his prostate cancer signature, a detailed description of his diagnosis and treatment to date. Then he began to tell his story:

"My wife Emily's sudden death in the summer of 1994 devastated me. It seemed impossible to go on, but there was no choice. The United Nations Volunteers asked me to produce a videotape of the work of two of their volunteers among the poor. The first volunteer was a pleasant Sri Lankan woman who did what a volunteer would typically do, teaching women how to make and market artificial flowers, cakes, and the like, extensions of the kitchen designed to keep women in their place. The other field worker was Gigi. She had enough going on in her slum area to require a couple of weeks of shooting, but I had allocated only two and a half days. Her projects were considered by some to be 'too assertive.' One involved arranging amnesty to give families who were illegal residents, who had come there to escape the poverty of diminishing farms, a chance to register legally. Then she began the process of getting birth certificates for their children, certificates that would allow them to attend school and begin life as productive citizens. Another project was to gather enough steel and to find the money to get cement to build a large garbage-composting center to give the impoverished community a source of income. I interviewed Gigi on camera for a couple of hours and I think that's when I began to love her. I was struck by her grasp of information, her logic, her gentleness, her vision—and her beauty."

Gigi replied: "Working with George was interesting because he listened to my opinions and thoughts. He was genuinely interested, a far cry from my husband, whom I left after fifteen years. Roberto was a womanizer who complained that I was 'always dry,' 'too loose down there' after my hysterectomy. He would force himself on me when drunk. When I couldn't take it anymore, I fled, shunning men and thinking they looked at women only as sex objects. When George and I first went to bed, he was so gentle. It was a strange feeling, and I was enjoying being touched. Finally, I had my first orgasm."

George continued: "It was around our third time

in bed together that Gigi began to relax enough to enjoy it. One day she asked me what an ejaculation felt like and I tried my best to tell her. She said 'That's what I had!' 'You had an orgasm,' I said. Then she told me. In fifteen years of being with Roberto she had never had an orgasm. This man, in addition to not supporting his family, misusing his employer's money, sleeping around and demeaning Gigi at every opportunity, had often raped her, usually while drunk, taking what he considered his with no regard ever for her pleasure."

The couple's sex life evolved: "At my age," George writes, "if I ejaculated when we had sex it could be two days before I could have intercourse again. So I learned to suggest we stop when I came close to orgasm. We'd stop and wait an hour or two, talking or sleeping or eating or whatever, then we'd make love again. I'd enjoy it thoroughly and Gigi would have another series of these waves of great orgasms. The continual lovemaking is very satisfying to me, and obviously to Gigi as well. I see stopping when close to orgasm as an act of love. I don't miss ejaculation, for I will always trade fifteen seconds of exquisite pleasure for the enduring pleasure of being the agent of Gigi's ecstasy."

The two were in love, but George's work took him far away again, to Armenia. He writes: "The Armenians are joyous people, and when I told them that my wife had died a few months before, they would not let me alone. They insisted that I should marry again, organized small dinners to work me over about it, prepared with food that was scarce and precious. One Sunday a young Armenian couple in love took me to the countryside, in the mountains in deep snow. They took me to a tiny chapel to light a candle for Emily. I got the message, lighting the candle in this remote place, with deep snow and strong wind and a loving couple as tour guides. It was a strange kind of closure. That night I faxed Gigi from my hotel, proposing marriage. Her reply the next day was 'Yes, yes!!' and then a few words to the effect of 'What took you so long?' "

Then George's cancer struck. He underwent a biopsy in France, when he developed urinary constriction and blood in his semen and after much consideration began combined hormonal blockade with Enantone (Leuproreline) and Anandron (Nilutamide), both forms of androgen ablation therapy or chemical castration. "The side effects were crippling," George writes. "Horrendous fatigue, lassitude, swelling and scabs on my lower legs, persistent depression finally neutralized by Zoloft and later St. John's Wort, a thirty-pound weight gain which meant I could no longer see my genitals. And loss of libido and erectile dysfunction."

Gigi and George weathered this period by exploring her sensitivity to kisses and caresses. Of this time, she wrote: "George's libido was almost zero. It was frustrating to both of us. I still had those waves of orgasms, but without his sexual enjoyment of them along with me, they were not the same."

The couple coped with his erectile dysfunction with a vacuum erection device (VED) known as the Osbon pump. George wrote; "The pump is a sophisticated piece of medical equipment, not a sex toy. It is sold by prescription and costs about $600, reimbursed 80% by my insurance. The pump creates an erection in a transparent hard plastic barrel. Gigi likes to manipulate it. She sits on me and creates designer erections, varying in size and texture according to her caprice. She seems to see me as a sort of yak." Gigi added: "We could only have sex with help of the pump, but we made it fun and interesting. The diagnosis made us scared, but we still had lots of sex."

Finally George's PSA test, which measures prostate-specific antigen, was low enough that he could begin intermittent anti-testosterone blockade, allowing his libido and erectile functioning to return almost to normal between doses. George wrote: "In my life before prostate cancer, I was impotent exactly three times, and these were once-only events, warnings by my body to keep the hell away from specific women. Now that I am impotent more often than not, I am not in despair, nor do I feel my manhood is threatened. But I do regret it. I do not believe that my impotence is good for our relationship, and we both enjoy intercourse most, but if there cannot be penetration because of the side effects of my treatment, so be it. We put other measures in place, but they are make-do measures at best. Gigi can stimulate me orally, which feels nice, or I can stimulate her. Closeness and kissing arouse her and give her an orgasm. That always astonishes me, but I refrain from laughing or chuckling with pleasure, for Gigi becomes embarrassed. This from a woman who didn't know what an orgasm was when we met."

George wrote: "My cancer is not organ confined. It had escaped the prostate capsule before it was diagnosed and was therefore inoperable. So it's still in there, dreaming of bone marrow but blocked from reaching it by the anti-androgens." George believes that the paucity of funds for prostate cancer research is related to the shame and secrecy of the diagnosis and the impotence that almost invariably accompanies its treatment.

So George and Gigi happy and in love, planning to marry (When, guys?) and awaiting Viagra's arrival, happy to hear of its 70% success rate from George's urologist, whom they visit regularly as a couple. They seem to know what really matters to them. Health, love, sex, and each other. For at least one couple on the planet, the verdict on Viagra is not yet in. But my sense is that whatever Viagra does or doesn't do for them, George and Gigi will be just fine.

If, as a psychiatrist, I could make Viagra do anything for all of us, it would be to make us appreciate that people, not pills, are what makes sex great. When the people involved are loving, pills can help make making love possible. If they're not, no pill in the world will help.

CONCLUSION

Sex is one of life's greatest pleasures, and with Viagra we have a chance to extend the length of time in our life spans that we can enjoy this fundamental aspect of our human-ness. We are the only animals who expect sex to go beyond reproduction, to be more than enough to ensure the survival of our kind. Sex can be the most intimate form of communication and expression of feelings, at whatever age and achieved through whatever means. Unlike those images in romance novels of young muscular studs with ever-hard penises and their always-wet-and-ready female mates, real love and sex take work and time. Those who know that lesson already or learn it before they take that first pill will ultimately be the ones Viagra helps most.

Acknowledgments

Deborah Wasser's contributions to this book were myriad and highly significant. She played a fundamental role in research for all aspects of the book. Her primary interviews with doctors and patients form the backbone of several chapters. We collaborated on the project from the start, shaping the concept and structure. Her humor and heart can be felt throughout as well, in style as well as content. Perhaps most significantly I credit Deb with infusing the subject with her spirit—her belief that sex is, as she'd say, our best little shot at ecstasy on this earth.

Thanks also to the many people who shared their stories with me, especially my patients and my on-line friends in the prostate cancer survivors support group. The courage, frankness, and strength of these men and their partners and families in the face of a dreadful disease is inspiring. A very special thanks to George and Gigi for sharing their story in their own words. I hope they will get their wish of increased attention and funding for men with prostate cancer.

My agent, Joy Harris, along with Kassandra Duane and Leslie Daniels, understood why I wanted to write

ACKNOWLEDGMENTS

this book from the start and worked hard to get it into the right hands. Mitchell Ivers, my editor at Pocket, helped me shape and hone the book at lightning speed, all the while maintaining a cheery demeanor and a sense of humor that helped me keep my center amid the whirlwind process. Thanks also to Amanda Ayers, Julie Blattberg, Donna O'Neill, Lisa Feuer, Joann Foster, Al Madocs, Allen Rosenblatt, and Jeff Theis for making it happen, and Emily Bestler and Gina Centrello for giving it a quick green light.

Thanks also to Jane Isay, who understood my desire for a torrid affair with Viagra and appreciated that it would not affect our "previous engagement," and to Steven Roose for giving me the time and space within my work schedule to do the project.

Last, but not least, thanks to Robert Glick for helping me to understand the true meaning of the phrase *carpe diem* and to act on it.